THE *"WORD"* ON HEALTH & NUTRITION

YOUR BODY GOD'S TEMPLE

From: *"The Word Works*-SELAH" series:

THE *"WORD"* ON HEALTH & NUTRITION

YOUR BODY GOD'S TEMPLE

by

JANNIE M. WILCOXSON

This book is not intended to provide medical advice. The nutritional and health information in this book is based on the teachings of the Word of God –the Bible-as well as research and personal experiences by the author. The publisher and author do not represent that the information in this book is to take the place of medical advice. Use of the information in this book is solely the responsibility and discretion of the reader. If you have questions regarding impact of diet, health, or exercise, you should speak to a health care physician.

Unless otherwise identified, all Scripture quotations are from the New American Standard Bible®, Copyright © 1960, 1962, 1963, 1968, 1971, 1972, 1973, 1975, 1977, 1995 by The Lockman Foundation. Used by permission.

Scripture references marked KJV are taken from the King James Version of the Bible.

Scripture quotations marked NKJV are taken from the New King James Version of the Bible. Copyright © 1982 by Thomas Nelson Inc. Used by permission. All rights reserved.

Cover design by Dwight David Quarmily

Published by: The Musicians Guild of America
Books & Music Publishing
3195 Dayton-Xenia Road
Suite 900 -107
Beavercreek, Ohio 45434

Printed in the United States of America

ISBN: 0-9792270-2-8

CONTENTS

Foreword

This book is written not to give you a list of dos and don'ts about what to eat. The emphasis is not on how bad certain foods are for you although a few are mentioned. It will not give you recipes or tell you how to plan a menu. It is not a medical journal but will give you some information from experts in the field of nutrition. What it will teach you is that if you are a believer, your body is the temple of the Holy Spirit and will guide you and cause you to walk in His statutes so that you honor God in <u>all things</u>. This book will open your eyes to what the Bible says about eating, its connection to obedience and how God has used food to test individuals throughout history. It will also encourage you to discipline your body and bring it into subjection so that you will live longer, healthier lives so that you will tell more people about Jesus.

This book will help you understand the whole counsel of the Word of God about our flesh and how to control it even in our eating habits. The flesh! Preachers preach on it, Churches teach on it and we have dealt with smoking, drugs, immorality, loving & hating one another, how to dress, drinking, gossip, etc., but we do not touch the eating habits of the body of Christ. Thank you for joining me in this study. If you are ready I am willing!

J. Wilcoxson

Psalms 107
20 He sent His word and healed them, And delivered them from their destructions.

Chapter 1

Christians Do Get Sick

> But you are a chosen race, a royal priesthood, a
> holy nation, a people for God's own possession, so
> that you may proclaim the excellencies of Him who
> has called you out of darkness into His marvelous
> light; 1 Peter 2:9

Have you ever wondered why Christians get sick like
everyone else? Why are we dying just like everyone else?
Why is our strength abated and eyes growing dim like
everyone else? Aren't we the ones who pray and God's
eyes are over the righteous so that He sees, hears, and
answers our prayers? Aren't we the called out ones, the
ekklesia, the church, the royal priesthood, the peculiar
people, the holy nation, the same ones God is calling for in
these last and evil days to be the light of the world and the
salt of the earth?

If the Bible is true, and it is, then why…why…why is the
Christian community so sick? Could it be that we are doing
what the world is doing in our eating habits, our exercise
habits, our sleep habits and other things that affect our
health?   Could it be that when we eat the standard
American diet (SAD) that we likewise experience the same
SAD results that the world experiences?   Lets go to the

Word of God and see what the Bible says about eating, about obedience, about health and about discipline.

Genesis 3 – This well-known chapter discusses the fall of man. Have you ever noticed that the fall of man is based on obedience, and the obedience is centered around "to eat" or "not to eat"? In Genesis 1 God created the heavens and earth, light, darkness as well as the sun, moon, stars, seas and dry land. Additionally God created living creatures on land, in the sea and in the air. He caused the earth to sprout vegetation and trees. Last of all God created man, planted a garden in Eden and placed man in this pre-planted garden to cultivate and keep it. Out of the ground, God caused to grow every tree that is pleasing to the sight and good for food. God created man in His own image and likeness; male and female He created them and gave them a few instructions:

1. Rule over the earth
2. Be fruitful, multiply, fill the earth, subdue it, & rule over every living thing that moves on the earth.
3. Adam was to cultivate and keep the garden.
4. Adam was told he could eat freely from any tree except the tree of knowledge of good and evil and if he would eat of it he would surely die (Gen 2:16-17) (*Notice the use of the word "eat"*)

Read Genesis 2:15-17 and underline the word *eat.*

> Genesis 2
> 15 Then the LORD God took the man and put him into the garden of Eden to cultivate it and keep it.
> 16 The LORD God commanded the man, saying, "From any tree of the garden you may eat freely;
> 17 but from the tree of the knowledge of good and evil you shall not eat, for in the day that you eat from it you will surely die."

2

Man has been told from Gen. 1:29 what his food was to be. Read Gen.1:29-30 and list what man can eat.

> Genesis 1
> 29 Then God said, "Behold, I have given you every plant yielding seed that is on the surface of all the earth, and every tree which has fruit yielding seed; it shall be food for you;
> 30 and to every beast of the earth and to every bird of the sky and to every thing that moves on the earth which has life, I have given every green plant for food"; and it was so.

Did you notice that man could not eat the animals and that the animals could not eat man?

Just so you can see for yourself, I have Gen.3 printed below. Read Gen.3:1-24 and simply underline the words *eat* or *ate*.

> Genesis 3
> 1 Now the serpent was more crafty than any beast of the field which the LORD God had made. And he said to the woman, "Indeed, has God said, 'You shall not eat from any tree of the garden'?"
> 2 The woman said to the serpent, "From the fruit of the trees of the garden we may eat;
> 3 but from the fruit of the tree which is in the middle of the garden, God has said, 'You shall not eat from it or touch it, or you will die.'"
> 4 The serpent said to the woman, "You surely will not die!
> 5 "For God knows that in the day you eat from it your eyes will be opened, and you will be like God, knowing good and evil."
> 6 When the woman saw that the tree was good for food, and that it was a delight to the eyes, and that the tree was desirable to make one wise, she took from its fruit and ate; and she gave also to her husband with her, and he ate.

7 Then the eyes of both of them were opened, and they knew that they were naked; and they sewed fig leaves together and made themselves loin coverings.

8 They heard the sound of the LORD God walking in the garden in the cool of the day, and the man and his wife hid themselves from the presence of the LORD God among the trees of the garden.

9 Then the LORD God called to the man, and said to him, "Where are you?"

10 He said, "I heard the sound of You in the garden, and I was afraid because I was naked; so I hid myself."

11 And He said, "Who told you that you were naked? Have you eaten from the tree of which I commanded you not to eat?"

12 The man said, "The woman whom You gave to be with me, she gave me from the tree, and I ate."

13 Then the LORD God said to the woman, "What is this you have done?" And the woman said, "The serpent deceived me, and I ate."

14 The LORD God said to the serpent, "Because you have done this, Cursed are you more than all cattle, And more than every beast of the field; On your belly you will go, And dust you will eat All the days of your life;

15 And I will put enmity Between you and the woman, And between your seed and her seed; He shall bruise you on the head, And you shall bruise him on the heel."

16 To the woman He said, "I will greatly multiply Your pain in childbirth, In pain you will bring forth children; Yet your desire will be for your husband, And he will rule over you."

17 Then to Adam He said, "Because you have listened to the voice of your wife, and have eaten from the tree about which I commanded you, saying, 'You shall not eat from it'; Cursed is the ground because of you; In toil you will eat of it All the days of your life.

18 "Both thorns and thistles it shall grow for you; And you will eat the plants of the field;

19 By the sweat of your face You will eat bread, Till you return to the ground, Because from it you were taken; For you are dust, And to dust you shall return."

20 Now the man called his wife's name Eve, because she was the mother of all the living.

21 The LORD God made garments of skin for Adam and his wife, and clothed them.

22 Then the LORD God said, "Behold, the man has become like one of Us, knowing good and evil; and now, he might stretch out his hand, and take also from the tree of life, and eat, and live forever" --

23 therefore the LORD God sent him out from the garden of Eden, to cultivate the ground from which he was taken.

24 So He drove the man out; and at the east of the garden of Eden He stationed the cherubim and the flaming sword which turned every direction to guard the way to the tree of life.

Repeated words in a passage are there to draw attention to something God wants us to see. While the main point of the passage is the fall of man, do not consider these repeated words as irrelevant to the text. How many times are the words *eat* and *ate* used? _____ What do we find?

The serpent enticed Eve to eat what she was told not to eat and promised that the result would provide something not normally received when eating food. The serpent appealed to the lust of the flesh, the lust of the eyes and the pride of life and Eve fell for it. She believed the lie and convinced Adam who was with her to eat of the tree. And he did! So Adam & Eve ate what they wanted instead of what God provided. Adam & Eve ate what they should not have eaten and they ate when they were not hungry and we have been doing the same thing every since!

They ate according to the serpent's promise that they would not die, that in fact they would be like God (Gen 3:4-5). I suppose they did not remember that they were created in the image and likeness of God.

What was the actual result of the fall of man (disobedience where food was used as a tool to entice Adam and Eve)?

- Adam & Eve hid from God
- Adam blamed Eve (although in Chapter 1 he called her 'bone of my bones and flesh of my flesh') and he also blamed God (*the blame game*)
- Eve admitted being deceived by the serpent, so she ate.
- God cursed the serpent
- God cursed the ground
- God clothed them with animal skins (*Notice the blood shed for them*)
- God put enmity between the seed of the woman and the serpent's seed. The serpent would bruise the heel of the woman's seed, but the woman's seed would bruise the head of the serpent's seed. (*Prophecy of the crucifixion-God solution for man's sin*)
- God said that pain in childbirth would multiply for the woman and her desire would be to her husband.
- God said the man would toil to eat from the ground, by the sweat of his brow (*remember God had placed them in a pre-planted luscious garden*).
- God said to dust you will return (*physical death*)
- God drove them out of the garden *(homeless)*

Verse 22 says (God is speaking) they have become like one of Us, knowing good and evil, but Adam and Eve received far more than they anticipated. As we look at the scripture and the results listed above, all of this because of one man's disobedience where food was used as a tool to entice, to test, to prove. Or shall we say because one man ate when he was not hungry, he ate something he should not have eaten, and he ate for the wrong motive. That sin took him further than he ever wanted to go. But that is not all, their disobedience went beyond that day and impacted more than Adam and Eve. Disobedience (eating the forbidden fruit) has impacted every person throughout the ages, every nation, every tribe and every tongue of in the entire world.

Look at this verse in Romans 5:12

> Romans 5
> 12 Therefore, just as through one man sin entered into the world, and death through sin, and so death spread to all men, because all sinned.

Do you see what happened? Sin entered the world and death through sin spread to all. Here is the good news.

> Romans 5
> 17 For if by the transgression of the one, death reigned through the one, much more those who receive the abundance of grace and of the gift of righteousness will reign in life through the One, Jesus Christ.
> 18 So then as through one transgression there resulted condemnation to all men, even so through one act of righteousness there resulted justification of life to all men.
> 19 For as through the one man's disobedience the many were made sinners, even so through the obedience of the One the many will be made righteous.

One man (Adam) bought death, but one man (Jesus) bought Life; one man (Adam) bought condemnation, but one man (Jesus) bought justification; one man (Adam) bought sin, but one man (Jesus) bought grace and righteousness. The fall of man that came about as a result of responding to the temptation of food was a fatal error, but the good news is that God through Jesus has an eternal solution! Have you got it yet?

Selah – Think about it!

1. What did man have the rule or authority over?

2. What is the key repeated word in Genesis 3?

3. At this point in scripture what is man's food?

4. What happened when Adam and Eve allowed their flesh to control their actions (in other words when they ate what they should not have eaten)?

5. Do you allow your flesh to control your actions? Do you eat when you are not hungry? Are you eating something you know you should not eat? How have your eating habits impacted others?

6. Have you believed Satan's lie (part truth is a whole lie) or will you believe all that God says about Himself and about you?

7. Why do you think Christians get sick like everyone else?

Chapter 2

Death Reigns, But God…Provides Life

> I will put none of the diseases on you…for I, the
> LORD, am your healer…(Exodus 15:26)

Psalm 90:10 promises 70 years of life, perhaps 80, and yet today humans are dying younger and younger; with the young experiencing the diseases of the old. Despite the advances of modern technology in medicines, state of the art equipment and numerous hospitals all over the world, many individuals never reach age 70 or beyond without experiencing devastating health problems in the last years of their lives. Why would that be? Why don't we see significant differences between the life span of Christians and everybody else?

We initially saw the death sentence of Adam and Eve experienced in Gen. 4 when Cain killed Abel; that was just the beginning. Just as God said, when we read Gen 5, we see the recording of their number of days, and their deaths "…and he died". By the time we reach chapter 6, the earth is evil continuously and God brings a flood on all the earth. In chapter 7 we see the mention of clean and unclean animals for the loading of the ark. After the flood, things changed significantly. Some believe there was a great change in the atmosphere and climate after the flood resulting in shorter life spans. Obviously *something* happened! Adam lived for 930 years, Noah lived for 500 years and Moses only lived for 120 years, but according to Deut. 34:7 his eye was not dim and his vigor not abated. (I know he walked and ate a lot of manna). There were other changes after the flood specifically in what could be eaten. Read Gen. 9:2-4, mark *eat* and *food* and notice what man could eat at this point.

> Genesis 9
> 2 "The fear of you and the terror of you will be on every beast of the earth and on every bird of the sky; with everything that creeps on the ground, and all the fish of the sea, into your hand they are given.
> 3 "Every moving thing that is alive shall be food for you; I give all to you, as I gave the green plant.
> 4 "Only you shall not eat flesh with its life, that is, its blood.

Did you get it? Man can now eat every moving thing that was alive. Don't get too excited there is more. They could not eat flesh with its life, that is, its blood. Oh well, so much for medium done or rare steak! Why would God give such instruction? For one thing during the flood, the waters covered the mountains, afterward God rebuked the waters, they fled, the mountains rose, the valleys sank and God sat a boundary that they (the waters) would never again cover the earth. (Psa. 104:6-9). In the meantime the results appear to have been a significant change in the earth, its climate and its vegetation. What about the blood? It is a well-known fact that blood carries infections and toxins that are in an animal's body. So could it be when people eat animal blood they are exposed to all the infections and toxins that the animals are carrying in their bodies?

Lets tie in another scripture from Exo.15. The children of Israel escaped from Egypt by way of the Red sea that God miraculously opened just for them and Moses' victory song is recorded. At the end of that chapter they have arrived at Marah and cannot drink the water because it is so bitter. So the people grumbled at Moses for water to drink seeming to forget that God just performed a miracle with water in the Red sea. Water was 'walled' up on each side as the children of Israel walked through. God showed Moses a tree, which he threw into the water and sweetened it. God made a statute and a regulation with them. Read the scripture below, marking what God said to them and what He required of them. Mark every verb!

> Exodus 15
> 26 And He said, "If you will give earnest heed to the voice of the LORD your God, and do what is right in His sight, and give ear to His commandments, and keep all His statutes, I will put none of the diseases on you which I have put on the Egyptians; for I, the LORD, am your healer."

God reveals Himself as Jehovah Rapha (I the LORD, am your healer). He says

if you…give earnest heed to the voice of the Lord (*listen*)

…do what is right in His sight (*do*)

…give ear to His commands (*listen*)

…keep all His statutes (*do*)

…then I will put none of these diseases on you

Word Study

Heal in Hebrew is *Rapha*, meaning "to mend (by stitching), i.e. (figuratively) to cure, (cause to) heal, physician, repair, thoroughly, make whole."

God's action is preventative, not after the fact! He promised to keep them healthy if they would obey. Obedience to the statutes to do what God says will heal, mend or repair. Obedience brings healing. Obedience was also the issue with Adam and Eve and here it is again. The scripture indicates that God had put the diseases on the Egyptians. Pathologist Marc A. Ruffer and others performed autopsies on mummies and found that the most common affliction of the Egyptians appears to be vascular diseases that resulted in calcified arteries (*this sounds like heart problems*). Other common diseases included arthritis, tooth decay, infections, cancer, emphysema, tuberculosis, parasites, pneumonia and obesity. The Pharaohs and royalty were the only ones whose diets included large quantities of meats and other delicacies (1 Kings 4:22 & Amos 6:4).

While the following verses do not mention eating, sickness and all forms of disease are promised for disobedience and the passage addresses what will happen to Israel if they chose not to obey.

> Deuteronomy 28
> 58 "If you are not careful to observe all the words of this law which are written in this book, to fear this honored and awesome name, the LORD your God,
> 59 then the LORD will bring extraordinary plagues on you and your descendants, even severe and lasting plagues, and miserable and chronic sicknesses.

60 "He will bring back on you all the diseases of Egypt of which you were afraid, and they will cling to you.

61 "Also every sickness and every plague which, not written in the book of this law, the LORD will bring on you until you are destroyed.

62 "Then you shall be left few in number, whereas you were as numerous as the stars of heaven, because you did not obey the LORD your God.

63 "It shall come about that as the LORD delighted over you to prosper you, and multiply you, so the LORD will delight over you to make you perish and destroy you; and you will be torn from the land where you are entering to possess it.

If they did not obey God would…

- Bring extraordinary plagues, severe, lasting, miserable and chronic sicknesses
- Bring back all the diseases of Egypt…and they will cling to you
- Bring every sicknesses and plague
- Make you perish and destroy you
- Tear you from the land

In Exodus after God reveals Himself as Jehovah-Rapha, lets see if Israel got the message. Read the following passage, record Israel's main concern and underline the word *ate*.

Exodus 16
1 Then they set out from Elim, and all the congregation of the sons of Israel came to the wilderness of Sin, which is between Elim and Sinai, on the fifteenth day of the second month after their departure from the land of Egypt.

2 The whole congregation of the sons of Israel grumbled against Moses and Aaron in the wilderness.

3 The sons of Israel said to them, "Would that we had died by the LORD'S hand in the land of Egypt, when we sat by the pots of meat, when we ate bread to the full; for you have brought us out into this wilderness to kill this whole assembly with hunger."

Israel grumbled less than two months after they left Egypt and their major concern is their hunger. They remember the food they ate, but not the misery inflicted on them by Pharaoh. They seemed to have forgotten that their lives were made bitter with hard, rigorous labor and very severe work conditions. They seemed to have forgotten that Egypt exercised population control by killing their boy babies and that God had delivered them from all those conditions. What Israel wanted and longed for was meat to eat like they had when they were in Egypt. But God is very compassionate, read on underlining God's solution and test for Israel; also circle *eat*.

Exodus 16
4 Then the LORD said to Moses, "Behold, I will rain bread from heaven for you; and the people shall go out and gather a day's portion every day, that I may test them, whether or not they will walk in My instruction.
5 "On the sixth day, when they prepare what they bring in, it will be twice as much as they gather daily."
6 So Moses and Aaron said to all the sons of Israel, "At evening you will know that the LORD has brought you out of the land of Egypt;
7 and in the morning you will see the glory of the LORD, for He hears your grumblings against the LORD; and what are we, that you grumble against us?"
8 Moses said, "This will happen when the LORD gives you meat to eat in the evening, and bread to the full in the morning; for the LORD hears your grumblings which you grumble against Him. And

what are we? Your grumblings are not against us but against the LORD."

9 Then Moses said to Aaron, "Say to all the congregation of the sons of Israel, 'Come near before the LORD, for He has heard your grumblings.'"

10 It came about as Aaron spoke to the whole congregation of the sons of Israel, that they looked toward the wilderness, and behold, the glory of the LORD appeared in the cloud.

11 And the LORD spoke to Moses, saying,

12 "I have heard the grumblings of the sons of Israel; speak to them, saying, 'At twilight you shall eat meat, and in the morning you shall be filled with bread; and you shall know that I am the LORD your God.'"

13 So it came about at evening that the quails came up and covered the camp, and in the morning there was a layer of dew around the camp.

14 When the layer of dew evaporated, behold, on the surface of the wilderness there was a fine flake-like thing, fine as the frost on the ground.

15 When the sons of Israel saw it, they said to one another, "What is it?" For they did not know what it was. And Moses said to them, "It is the bread which the LORD has given you to eat.

God in His compassion provided meat for Israel. He also provided bread. Please read on, marking the instructions God gives Israel and circle the word *eat*.

Exodus

16 "This is what the LORD has commanded, 'Gather of it every man as much as he should eat; you shall take an omer apiece according to the number of persons each of you has in his tent.'"

17 The sons of Israel did so, and some gathered much and some little.

18 When they measured it with an omer, he who had gathered much had no excess, and he who had gathered little had no lack; every man gathered as much as he should eat.

19 Moses said to them, "Let no man leave any of it until morning."

20 But they did not listen to Moses, and some left part of it until morning, and it bred worms and became foul; and Moses was angry with them.

21 They gathered it morning by morning, every man as much as he should eat; but when the sun grew hot, it would melt.

22 Now on the sixth day they gathered twice as much bread, two omers for each one. When all the leaders of the congregation came and told Moses,

23 then he said to them, "This is what the LORD meant: Tomorrow is a sabbath observance, a holy sabbath to the LORD. Bake what you will bake and boil what you will boil, and all that is left over put aside to be kept until morning."

24 So they put it aside until morning, as Moses had ordered, and it did not become foul nor was there any worm in it.

25 Moses said, "Eat it today, for today is a sabbath to the LORD; today you will not find it in the field.

26 "Six days you shall gather it, but on the seventh day, the sabbath, there will be none."

27 It came about on the seventh day that some of the people went out to gather, but they found none.

28 Then the LORD said to Moses, "How long do you refuse to keep My commandments and My instructions?

The instructions were:
- Gather as much as they could eat
- None was to be left until morning
- On day 6 gather enough food for 2 days

What they did:
- Some left part until morning, it bred worms
- On Day 6 they did not gather 2 days worth of food but went out on day 7 to gather and found nothing

Read the following scriptures and write down the name of the bread.

Exodus 16

29 "See, the LORD has given you the sabbath; therefore He gives you bread for two days on the sixth day. Remain every man in his place; let no man go out of his place on the seventh day."

30 So the people rested on the seventh day.

31 The house of Israel named it manna, and it was like coriander seed, white, and its taste was like wafers with honey.

One more verse – Read verse 35 – how long did Israel eat manna? Circle the word *ate*.

Exodus 16

35 The sons of Israel ate the manna forty years, until they came to an inhabited land; they ate the manna until they came to the border of the land of Canaan.

Isn't it interesting that Israel complained and grumbled against Moses about food and they did not seem to trust God enough to follow the simple rules of how much manna to gather, when to gather it, and when to keep leftovers. Once again they fail the test of obedience preferring to return to Egypt for the food (actually the return would be to bondage) rather than to obey God. You will also remember that food was the tool that lead to the disobedience of Adam and Eve. They chose the Serpent's plan rather than to follow God's simple rule not to eat of the tree in the middle of the garden.

Selah –Think about it

1. When was man permitted to eat meat?

2. When did the lifespan of man begin to shorten?

3. What diseases did God promise not to put on Israel and what were the conditions?

4. What is the connection between obedience, health and healing?

5. Why do you think Christians get sick like everyone else?

Chapter 3

Is God's power limited?

"Is the LORD'S power limited? Now you shall see whether My word will come true for you or not." Num 11:23

Are you stuck? Stuck where food is controlling you? Stuck where your appetite or desire exceeds your will to obey, especially when you know what is right and what you should do. So stuck that you make poor eating choices that affect your health, happiness, longevity of life and even the lives of those around you. What can you do and how do you get relief when you get stuck in an area of disobedience? As we continue to study the life of Israel we find some excellent examples so that through perseverance and encouragement of the scriptures, we can have hope.

Escaped from Egypt a few months earlier, Israel is well on their way to the promised land. The camp arrangement of the tribes has been made, the people are numbered for battle, and the duties of the Levites have been clearly defined. One thing that was consistent among the group was their complaints. Read Numbers 11:4-6 and record their most recent compliant. Circle *eat*.

Numbers 11

4 The rabble who were among them had greedy desires; and also the sons of Israel wept again and said, "Who will give us meat to eat?

5 "We remember the fish which we used to eat free in Egypt, the cucumbers and the melons and the leeks and the onions and the garlic,

6 but now our appetite is gone. There is nothing at all to look at except this manna."

Israel has been eating manna in many different forms and ways for 40 years. They would grind it, beat it, boil it, make cakes with it and they were very tired of manna even though it had sustained them all these years. It was like left over thanksgiving dinner, bake it, boil it, make a salad, or barbeque it just to eat it a different way. It was good the first day, but after a while it gets pretty old. Read on.

Numbers 11

10 Now Moses heard the people weeping throughout their families, each man at the doorway of his tent; and the anger of the LORD was kindled greatly, and Moses was displeased.

11 So Moses said to the LORD, "Why have You been so hard on Your servant? And why have I not found favor in Your sight, that You have laid the burden of all this people on me?

12 "Was it I who conceived all this people? Was it I who brought them forth, that You should say to me, 'Carry them in your bosom as a nurse carries a nursing infant, to the land which You swore to their fathers'?

13 "Where am I to get meat to give to all this people? For they weep before me, saying, 'Give us meat that we may eat!'

14 "I alone am not able to carry all this people, because it is too burdensome for me.

15 "So if You are going to deal thus with me, please kill me at once, if I have found favor in Your sight, and do not let me see my wretchedness."

They are stuck! The people are weeping, the men standing in their doorways are weeping. God is angry and Moses is displeased – the surface problem is that Israel wants food from Egypt. The underlying problem is that the people are ungrateful not only for God's provision of food, but also for their release from bondage in Egypt. Moses, knowing that God is sovereign, is so distraught that God would allow such a burden to fall on him. Remember the problem is that the people want to eat and Moses is burdened to provide for them. At this point in Israel's history there are over 600,000 men not including women and children that must be cared for. Moses reminds God that he did not conceive them or nurse them and felt it was too much for him to bear. Have you ever felt that a situation that you have been in was too difficult to bear and have you ever wanted to scream "I just can't take it." It is so amazing that this food issue has so distressed Moses that he desires to die especially if God is going to continue to deal with him with such a heavy burden. It has become a very devastating situation and often is when you deal with folks and food. You may be thinking-what is the big deal, they just want some good tasty food. God tells us the real problem in verses 18-20 and of course He has a solution. Read on, marking God's plan as you read. Circle *eat*.

Numbers 11
16 The LORD therefore said to Moses, "Gather for Me seventy men from the elders of Israel, whom you know to be the elders of the people and their officers and bring them to the tent of meeting, and let them take their stand there with you.
17 "Then I will come down and speak with you there, and I will take of the Spirit who is upon you, and will put Him upon them; and they shall bear the

burden of the people with you, so that you will not bear it all alone.

18 "Say to the people, 'Consecrate yourselves for tomorrow, and you shall eat meat; for you have wept in the ears of the LORD, saying, "Oh that someone would give us meat to eat! For we were well-off in Egypt." Therefore the LORD will give you meat and you shall eat.

19 'You shall eat, not one day, nor two days, nor five days, nor ten days, nor twenty days,

20 but a whole month, until it comes out of your nostrils and becomes loathsome to you; because you have rejected the LORD who is among you and have wept before Him, saying, "Why did we ever leave Egypt?"'"

So God is going to provide food, but He is angry because they have rejected Him and they are willing to go back into bondage just for a piece of meat and a slice of cucumber. They said 'we were well off in Egypt', but God calls out their real problem. Are there foods that have put you in or kept you in bondage because of a lack of discipline? Bondages that have led to obesity, lack of energy, sicknesses, laziness, greed, addictions and compulsions? Be careful what you ask for. Initially, it appears that God gives them exactly what they want. But what they want and deeply desire will lead to something they never anticipated when they rejected God, His provisions and His standard. God will feed them and they will eat until it comes out of their noses. This is also a great lesson for Moses who cannot see how God will provide food for so many people.

Numbers 11

21 But Moses said, "The people, among whom I am, are 600,000 on foot; yet You have said, 'I will give them meat, so that they may eat for a whole month.'

22 "Should flocks and herds be slaughtered for them, to be sufficient for them? Or should all the fish of the sea be gathered together for them, to be sufficient for them?"

24

23 The LORD said to Moses, "Is the LORD'S power limited? Now you shall see whether My word will come true for you or not."

When you are stuck that's a word to be embraced, "is the Lord's power limited?" Take that one and put it in any situation of your life, stuck or not. Moses followed God's instruction and called the elders to help in this burden bearing, food-handling situation and God begins to work. Did you notice that God does not remove the problem, but He provides help? Read the rest of the story looking for God's provision and the people's response. Write it out below:

Numbers 11
31 Now there went forth a wind from the LORD and it brought quail from the sea, and let them fall beside the camp, about a day's journey on this side and a day's journey on the other side, all around the camp and about two cubits deep on the surface of the ground.
32 The people spent all day and all night and all the next day, and gathered the quail (he who gathered least gathered ten homers) and they spread them out for themselves all around the camp.
33 While the meat was still between their teeth, before it was chewed, the anger of the LORD was kindled against the people, and the LORD struck the people with a very severe plague.
34 So the name of that place was called Kibroth-hattaavah, because there they buried the people who had been greedy.

God's provision

People's response:

God struck the people with a plague. It was while the meat was still between their teeth that God's anger was kindled against them. Read verse 34 again, people die and are buried because of greed. Not only do they reject God, but they are greedy and it kills them. This reminds me of all the diseases that have come upon people today because of greed or uncontrolled desire of multitudes that have eaten something that has caused or lead to their deaths. Israel had a tough time getting Egypt out of their systems and over and over again they tried the Lord with their complaining, impatience, and grumbling. While the Lord's power is not limited, He may choose not to use His power to deliver us in the way we may want Him to. God is not trying to conform to us, we are to conform to God. Israel desperately needs to learn this lesson of obedience. God wants to move them to a higher level of obedience. When we do not obey in small, basic areas, how do we think we can obey when the larger tasks, responsibilities and assignments come? Soon God is going to take Israel to the promised land of Canaan (Num 13), they are simply to go in and take the land. They do not do it and wander in the wilderness for 40 years because they have not learned obedience. Is there an area of obedience you need to work on so that God can move you to another level of growth and victory?

Read the following passage and underline their complaint. Circle *food*.

> Numbers 21
> 4 Then they set out from Mount Hor by the way of the Red Sea, to go around the land of Edom; and the people became impatient because of the journey.

5 The people spoke against God and Moses, "Why have you brought us up out of Egypt to die in the wilderness? For there is no food and no water, and we loathe this miserable food."

The people speak against God and Moses. Not a well thought out action. Speaking against the One who provides their food, whose earth they are walking on, whose roof they are walking under and whose air they are breathing can only lead to trouble with Elohim (Creator God). The miserable food that they loathed was the manna God provided for them and that had sustained them for forty years. Once again the issue involves food and water. It is amazing how the flesh continues to crave the very thing that can kill it. God's response is to send in fiery serpents and many people die. Suddenly the people 'get it' or at least they acknowledge their sin of speaking against the Lord. Read the passage below and underline their response and request to Moses.

Numbers 21
6 The LORD sent fiery serpents among the people and they bit the people, so that many people of Israel died.
7 So the people came to Moses and said, "We have sinned, because we have spoken against the LORD and you; intercede with the LORD, that He may remove the serpents from us." And Moses interceded for the people.

How quickly they realize their error when people begin to die. Immediately they turn to Moses and ask him to pray for them. Moses, faithful & true to God, intercedes for the people. Read on for God's surprising response.

Numbers 21
8 Then the LORD said to Moses, "Make a fiery serpent, and set it on a standard; and it shall come

about, that everyone who is bitten, when he looks at
it, he will live."
9 And Moses made a bronze serpent and set it on
the standard; and it came about, that if a serpent bit
any man, when he looked to the bronze serpent, he
lived.

Surprise! Enough is enough! God does not remove the
serpents. Can you believe it? God has the power to
remove these serpents, but chooses not to. Instead He
instructs Moses to make a bronze serpent. (Bronze serpent
– Mmmm, wonder if this is where the medical community
got the idea of their 'serpent' symbol?) When the people
that have been bitten by the serpents looked on this bronze
serpent they would live. Want to know what to do when
you are stuck in disobedience? Read that passage
carefully! In order to be healed and live, dying people had
to follow instructions, they had to obey God, they had to
look up to live. Do you see that God uses this occasion of
the people complaining about food and water to provide
them the opportunity to change their lives by obedience?
To change from the state of dying to that of living! In John
3 when Jesus is talking to Nicodemus about what it means
to be born again, He refers to this same passage. This is
what He said in John 3:14.

John 3
14 "As Moses lifted up the serpent in the
wilderness, even so must the Son of Man be lifted
up;
15 so that whoever believes will in Him have
eternal life.

When Jesus is lifted up He will draw all men to Himself
giving those who are infected and dying to sin an
opportunity to look to Jesus, believe, be healed, saved and
to live for an eternity. Numbers 11 and Numbers 21 is
more than about food, but once again food is used as the
test vehicle. It is much deeper when you think that Israel is

ungrateful for God's deliverance, they are rejecting God's provision and protection, they are disobedient, they are greedy, and they are desiring to go back into a bondage situation just for food. Over and over you hear the complaints of the people about food and water and over and over again you see God providing the opportunity for the people to live by obedience. If they do not get it today, if they do not learn obedience today, how will they obey tomorrow? Can you relate to what Israel is experiencing? Are you stuck? Will you take a real good look at how this may impact your life and the lives of others?

Selah – think about it

1. Why is God so angry with Israel? What is their specific area of disobedience? Are you learning to obey?

2. How does the desire of the flesh keep you from being obedient to God?   Are you stuck in some area of disobedience, food or otherwise?

3. Why is Moses asking God to kill him rather than burden him with this food problem?

4. What did you learn about food and how it can control your actions?

5. Make a list of bondages that you are aware of in your life and how you can break them.

6. What did you learn about God in these chapters?

Why do you think Christians get sick like everyone else?

Chapter 4

Breaking Addictions - Fasting

> "Is this not the fast which I choose, To loosen the bonds of wickedness, To undo the bands of the yoke, And to let the oppressed go free And break every yoke?" Isaiah 58:6

What do we do with the cravings of the flesh? How do we bring our uncontrolled appetites of the flesh into submission? These appetites are very dangerous to our health and well-being and must be controlled. As you study the scriptures below you will see how a spiritual problem can manifest itself physically in our bodies. Fasting is a powerful discipline that can help us bring uncontrolled appetites into submission.

Word Study

Fasting in Hebrew is *tsuwm* meaning "to cover over (the mouth)".

Fasting in Greek it is *nestis* meaning "to abstain from food."

It is reasonable to think that abstinence from food would have a physical effect on our bodies, and it does. God made the human body to heal itself. So when we fast our bodies eliminate poisons and toxins, which promotes self-healing and provides the body the opportunity to rejuvenate itself. It seems to go beyond human reasoning to think that abstinence from food would also have a significant effect spiritually, mentally, emotionally, and psychologically. Read the following scripture to see the benefits of fasting. In this passage of scripture the Israelites have fasted and are wondering why God does not see what they are doing so as to respond to what they want from Him.

> Isaiah 58
> 3 'Why have we fasted and You do not see? Why have we humbled ourselves and You do not notice?' Behold, on the day of your fast you find your desire, And drive hard all your workers.
> 4 "Behold, you fast for contention and strife and to strike with a wicked fist. You do not fast like you do today to make your voice heard on high.

God told Israel that they were fasting for the following reasons:

To find their desire
They are driving their workers
For contention and strife
They are not fasting to make their voices heard on high

God outlines the fast He desires. Mark the reasons as you read.

> Isaiah 58
> 5 "Is it a fast like this which I choose, a day for a man to humble himself? Is it for bowing one's head like a reed And for spreading out sackcloth and ashes as a bed? Will you call this a fast, even an acceptable day to the LORD?

God lets them know that the fast is not just a matter of externally afflicting yourself, of bowing the head and spreading sackcloth and ashes, but it should be acceptable to the Lord. Fasting should impact their lives and the lives of others around them, treatment of others and attitudes will change. It is done not to be seen of men but to be acceptable to the Lord. Continue to mark the reasons for fasting as you read.

> Isaiah 58
> 6 "Is this not the fast which I choose, To loosen the bonds of wickedness, To undo the bands of the yoke, And to let the oppressed go free And break every yoke?
> 7 "Is it not to divide your bread with the hungry And bring the homeless poor into the house; When you see the naked, to cover him; And not to hide yourself from your own flesh?

Benefits:
- o To humble yourself
- o Bowing the head
- o Spread out sackcloth and ashes
- o Acceptable to the Lord
- o Loosen the bonds of wickedness
- o Undo the bands of the yoke
- o Let the oppressed go free
- o Break every yoke
- o Divide your bread with the hungry
- o Bring the homeless poor into the house
- o Cover the naked
- o Not to hide yourself

After the fast what does God promise?   More benefits!
Mark them as you read. Don't miss the healing.

Isaiah 58
8 "Then your light will break out like the dawn,
And your recovery will speedily spring forth; And
your righteousness will go before you; The glory of
the
9 "Then you will call, and the LORD will answer;
You will cry, and He will say, 'Here I am.' If you
remove the yoke from your midst, The pointing of
the finger and speaking wickedness,
10 And if you give yourself to the hungry And
satisfy the desire of the afflicted, Then your light
will rise in darkness And your gloom will become
like midday.
11 "And the LORD will continually guide you,
And satisfy your desire in scorched places, And
give strength to your bones; And you will be like a
watered garden, And like a spring of water whose
waters do not fail.

More Benefits:
  o   Your light will break forth
  o   Your recovery will speedily spring forth
  o   Your righteousness will go before you
  o   The glory of the lord will be your rearguard
  o   You call-God answers
  o   You cry – God is there
  o   You remove the yoke, pointing finger, speaking
       wickedness & give yourself to the
  o   hungry and then your light will rise in darkness
  o   Your gloom will come like midday
  o   The Lord will continually guide you
  o   God will satisfy you in scorched places
  o   God will give strength to your bones
  o   You will be like a watered garden and a spring that
       does not fail

Go back and put a checkmark by the benefits you really want to see in your life. When you fast as God desires you will turn from doing your own pleasures and from seeking your own pleasure and from speaking your own word, but instead you will take delight in the Lord. Are you willing?

It is interesting to see what happens when we abstain from food (fast) with the right attitude and how God responds. Look for and record why the individuals were fasting and how God responded.

Ezra 8
21 Then I proclaimed a fast there at the river of Ahava, that we might humble ourselves before our God to seek from Him a safe journey for us, our little ones, and all our possessions.
22 For I was ashamed to request from the king troops and horsemen to protect us from the enemy on the way, because we had said to the king, "The hand of our God is favorably disposed to all those who seek Him, but His power and His anger are against all those who forsake Him."
23 So we fasted and sought our God concerning this matter, and He listened to our entreaty.

Why were they fasting? What was God's response? From verse 22 what do you know about God and those who seek Him?

Jonah 3
5 Then the people of Nineveh believed in God; and they called a fast and put on sackcloth from the greatest to the least of them.

35

6 When the word reached the king of Nineveh, he arose from his throne, laid aside his robe from him, covered himself with sackcloth and sat on the ashes.

7 He issued a proclamation and it said, "In Nineveh by the decree of the king and his nobles: Do not let man, beast, herd, or flock taste a thing. Do not let them eat or drink water.

8 "But both man and beast must be covered with sackcloth; and let men call on God earnestly that each may turn from his wicked way and from the violence which is in his hands.

9 "Who knows, God may turn and relent and withdraw His burning anger so that we will not perish."

10 When God saw their deeds, that they turned from their wicked way, then God relented concerning the calamity which He had declared He would bring upon them. And He did not do it.

Why were they fasting? What action did they take? What was God's response?

Psalm 35

13 But as for me, when they were sick, my clothing was sackcloth; I humbled my soul with fasting, And my prayer kept returning to my bosom.

Why the fast? What action was taken? What was God's response?

Esther 4

16 "Go, assemble all the Jews who are found in Susa, and fast for me; do not eat or drink for three days, night or day. I and my maidens also will fast in the same way. And thus I will go in to the king, which is not according to the law; and if I perish, I perish."

In this instance Esther called a corporate fast by the Jewish community when the evil prime minister of Persia (Haman) was successful in passing a law that would require the lives of all the Jews. Esther decided to risk her life by going before the king to save her people from this death sentence. So Esther went before the king dressed in her royal robes (not sackcloth and ashes, by the way). She invited the King to dinner along with the evil Haman. Haman's plot was exposed and as he begged for mercy, the king thought he was making a play for his wife, Esther. Haman was hanged on the gallows he had prepared for Mordecai (Esther's cousin) and the Jews were saved. Why the fast? The fast was for protection for Esther as she approached the king, for favor from God in every area and for deliverance for all the Jews from the death sentence. What a mighty move of God we see in this story as God works on behalf of His people.

> Psalm 109
> 24 My knees are weak from fasting, And my flesh has grown lean, without fatness.

What happened while the psalmist was fasting?

> Acts 13
> 1 Now there were at Antioch, in the church that was there, prophets and teachers: Barnabas, and Simeon who was called Niger, and Lucius of Cyrene, and Manaen who had been brought up with Herod the tetrarch, and Saul.
> 2 While they were ministering to the Lord and fasting, the Holy Spirit said, "Set apart for Me Barnabas and Saul for the work to which I have called them."
> 3 Then, when they had fasted and prayed and laid their hands on them, they sent them away.

Why were they fasting? What other action did they take?
What was God's response?

Matthew 17
15 "Lord, have mercy on my son, for he is a lunatic
and is very ill; for he often falls into the fire and
often into the water.
16 "I brought him to Your disciples, and they could
not cure him."
17 And Jesus answered and said, "You unbelieving
and perverted generation, how long shall I be with
you? How long shall I put up with you? Bring him
here to Me."
18 And Jesus rebuked him, and the demon came
out of him, and the boy was cured at once.
19 Then the disciples came to Jesus privately and
said, "Why could we not drive it out?"
20 And He *said to them, "Because of the littleness
of your faith; for truly I say to you, if you have faith
the size of a mustard seed, you will say to this
mountain, 'Move from here to there,' and it will
move; and nothing will be impossible to you.
21 "But this kind does not go out except by prayer
and fasting."

Why was there a need for fasting? What other actions
should be added to the fasting?

Daniel 10
1 In the third year of Cyrus king of Persia a
message was revealed to Daniel, who was named
Belteshazzar; and the message was true and one of
great conflict, but he understood the message and
had an understanding of the vision.
2 In those days, I, Daniel, had been mourning for
three entire weeks.

3 I did not eat any tasty food, nor did meat or wine enter my mouth, nor did I use any ointment at all until the entire three weeks were completed.

Daniel is fasting! Underline what he does not eat in verse 3. How long was the fast?

Daniel 10
12 Then he said to me, "Do not be afraid, Daniel, for from the first day that you set your heart on understanding this and on humbling yourself before your God, your words were heard, and I have come in response to your words.
13 "But the prince of the kingdom of Persia was withstanding me for twenty-one days; then behold, Michael, one of the chief princes, came to help me, for I had been left there with the kings of Persia.
14 "Now I have come to give you an understanding of what will happen to your people in the latter days, for the vision pertains to the days yet future."

Why was Daniel fasting? What was God's response? When did God hear Daniel and why was it so long before Daniel received the answer?

There was another time that Daniel fasted at the beginning of his captivity. Daniel and three young men (Shadrach, Meshach and Abednego) were captured by the Babylonians and taken from their country, their family and their culture. They were the top of the crop in that they were well educated, good-looking and very well endowed in wisdom, understanding and knowledge. They were to be educated in the ways of the Chaldeans so they could eventually enter the king's service. The king chose their food. Read on.

Daniel 1
5 The king appointed for them a daily ration from the king's choice food and from the wine which he drank, and appointed that they should be educated

three years, at the end of which they were to enter the king's personal service.

Daniel chose not to partake of the king's food. No doubt he knew the Jewish dietary laws and the requirements God had set forth for his people. Read on for Daniel's response and what God did for him.

> Daniel 1
> 8 But Daniel made up his mind that he would not defile himself with the king's choice food or with the wine which he drank; so he sought permission from the commander of the officials that he might not defile himself.
> 9 Now God granted Daniel favor and compassion in the sight of the commander of the officials,
> 10 and the commander of the officials said to Daniel, "I am afraid of my lord the king, who has appointed your food and your drink; for why should he see your faces looking more haggard than the youths who are your own age? Then you would make me forfeit my head to the king."

Daniel is very respectful in his request. However, the commander of the officials is concerned that if Daniel does not do what everyone else does, he will look haggard. The commander's response is much like ours today. Of course a major reason is that he did not want to lose his head. With all due respect, Daniel makes a deal with the commander so that he and his friends become the test group for 10 days. Read on and underline what they agree to eat, and the test results.

> Daniel 1
> 11 But Daniel said to the overseer whom the commander of the officials had appointed over Daniel, Hananiah, Mishael and Azariah,
> 12 "Please test your servants for ten days, and let us be given some vegetables to eat and water to drink.
> 13 "Then let our appearance be observed in your presence and the appearance of the youths who are

40

eating the king's choice food; and deal with your servants according to what you see."

14 So he listened to them in this matter and tested them for ten days.

15 At the end of ten days their appearance seemed better and they were fatter than all the youths who had been eating the king's choice food.

16 So the overseer continued to withhold their choice food and the wine they were to drink, and kept giving them vegetables.

Obviously Daniel knew something about healthy eating and made a decision based on what he knew.

Word Study

<u>Vegetables</u> in Hebrew is *zeroa* or *zeraSon* meaning "something sown, i.e. a vegetable (as food)-pulse."

This consisted of vegetables, grains, wheat, barley, rye, peas, beans and lentils. This means they did eat, but eliminated all the tempting rich food from the king's table, meats, cakes, pies, pastries and wine. Not only do they know what to eat, they obviously have favor with God. Read on looking for how these young men turned out.

Daniel 1

17 As for these four youths, God gave them knowledge and intelligence in every branch of literature and wisdom; Daniel even understood all kinds of visions and dreams.

18 Then at the end of the days which the king had specified for presenting them, the commander of the officials presented them before Nebuchadnezzar.

19 The king talked with them, and out of them all not one was found like Daniel, Hananiah, Mishael and Azariah; so they entered the king's personal service.

20 As for every matter of wisdom and understanding about which the king consulted them, he found them ten times better than all the magicians and conjurers who were in all his realm.

Verse 20 is the result of the three-year preparation period and the vegetarian diet they were consuming. They were presented to the king to enter into service and they were found to be ten times better than everyone else. Do you think the way they turned out (10 times better than all...) had anything to do with what they were eating? Do you think their thinking had anything to do with what they were eating? Wonder why God included this passage in His inspired Word?

Lets summarize! Although we did not look at every passage on fasting in this book, without exception in the Bible when people fasted, prayed and repented God released His supernatural power in their lives. Some reasons for and results of fasting that we found in the scriptures we studied:

- Isa. 58   -Loosen the bonds of wickedness, break yokes, speedy recovery + much more
- Ezra 8   -Direction and protection
- Jonah 3 -God's favor and to overcome wickedness
- Psa. 35   -Humble the soul
- Psa. 109 -Knees weak and flesh lean
- Est. 4   -Direction, divine favor and protection
- Acts 13   -Set apart and sent out for God's work
- Matt. 17 -For empowered ministry
- Dan. 1   -To overcome the flesh
- Dan. 10 -Spiritual breakthrough-humility & understanding

Can you believe it? Abstain from food, push away from the table, turn down your plate and what incredible benefits we see from fasting. Do it God's way and you will not just walk away hungry, but you will walk away spiritually enriched.

Selah – think about it

1. What in the world does fasting have to do with our physical health?

2. What significant changes can happen in our spiritual health as we fast?

3. How does fasting help control our fleshy appetites? Do I want to fulfill my appetites or do I want to fulfill God's will?

4. How does fasting break addictions?

5. What are some benefits of fasting?

6. What kind of fast does God require?

7. Can you see why Christians get sick like everyone else?

8. For extra study on fasting, see the following scriptures:

Scripture	Why Fast	Results
1 Sam 7:3-14		
2 Sam 1:12		
2 Sam 12:13-23		
1 Kings 21:20-29		
Neh 1:1-2:6		
Psalm 69:6-13		
Jere 14:10-17		
Zech 7		
Dan 9:1-6		
Mk 4:1-11		
Lk 5:30-35		
Acts 14:23		

Holy Spirit, Thou take over
Break me from this binding foe
Clean me, build me, make me free
Your healing touch I'll know.

Give me strength to beat my flesh
To look the other way
To deny myself and cling to you
To do exactly what YOU say.

E. Ward

Chapter 5

Prayer and Your Health

"But for you who fear My name, the sun of righteousness will rise with healing in its wings; and you will go forth and skip about like calves from the stall. (Mal. 4:2)

How do we pray with confidence about our health? When you have the report of disease in your body or you are always tired, have little or no energy, your skin is shallow, your hair is lifeless, your eyes are dim and you have difficulty focusing, always distracted and restless, what will prayer do? When your physical condition affects your mental and your emotional state and vice versa, how can you confidently approach God in prayer and expect to get an answer? When you have prayed and prayed and you cannot seem to hear from God, how do you get a prayer through? Have you resigned yourself to live in the state you are in or will you seek God's face?

It is the humble and contrite heart that is totally dependant on God that runs with confidence to the throne of grace. The result is a deeper relationship with God. What is the confidence we can have? Read 1 John 5:14-15 and underline how we can be sure to get an answer?

1 John 5

14 This is the confidence which we have before Him, that, if we ask anything according to His will, He hears us.

15 And if we know that He hears us in whatever we ask, we know that we have the requests which we have asked from Him.

What a wonderful assurance to know that God will hear and answer our prayers when we pray in accordance with His will. Not only will He hear, but we can know that when it is according to his will we have what we ask.

Read the next verse and underline what God expects from His people and His promise.

2 Chronicles 7

14 and My people who are called by My name humble themselves and pray and seek My face and turn from their wicked ways, then I will hear from heaven, will forgive their sin and will heal their land.

God expects His people to:
    Humble themselves
    Pray
    Seek His face
    Turn from their wicked ways

God promises to:
    Hear
    Forgive the sin
    Heal the land

That is what God expects from *His people*. He does not expect this from those who are not His. So He is not waiting for the world to change before He heals the land, He is waiting for His people to obey and then He will heal the land. Humble people, praying people seeking God's face, repentant people, forgiven people, healed people, healed land! Can you see why the land is not healed? Obviously God is talking specifically to Israel, but we can see the sinful state of our country today and know that God will heal our land when we follow the same example of obedience.

The prayer becomes very personal as we ask ourselves why our land is not healed? Is it because I am not doing my part? Have I prayed? Have I sought His face? Have I turned from my wicked ways? Am I walking in forgiveness of sin? Is the land healed? Am I healed, physically, mentally, emotionally, spiritually? Can I help someone else walk in God's healing? Many of the people of God have not, will not, cannot and basically do not handle personal issues or other relational issues very well. Unfortunately when we do not handle our own personal issues, these unresolved problems affect how we handle everything and how we relate to others.

Handling Issues.

This is a major problem that impacts our health when we do not handle issues on a daily basis. Good eating habits will do little when there is a spiritual issue that needs to be handled. These issues could be at home, on the job, in the marketplace, at school, at church or in the community. Finances, relationships, communication, self-esteem, pride, or anything that leads you away from the Word of God and how He tells us to live. When you do not deal with these spiritual issues you will experience physical, mental & emotional trauma and everyone else around you feels the impact. Issues left unmanaged will change your personality, impact your integrity, could damage your character and your health if not handled expeditiously.

The following passage shows what happens when an issue surfaces, how it is handled, who is affected and how the power of prayer works in this situation. Read the passage and identify the problem by underlining it.

> Numbers 12
> 1 Then Miriam and Aaron spoke against Moses because of the Cushite woman whom he had married (for he had married a Cushite woman);
> 2 and they said, "Has the LORD indeed spoken only through Moses? Has He not spoken through us as well?" And the LORD heard it.
> 3 (Now the man Moses was very humble, more than any man who was on the face of the earth.)

The problem Miriam & Aaron have with Moses is two-fold. They have a problem with his wife and they have a problem with the authority God has given him. His two siblings do not say what problem they have with his wife except that she is a foreigner. Although they challenge his leadership, they both know how and when God called Moses as well as when God called them. They both had clear and specific assignments, but they question Moses. Moses does not answer a word. Read and underline what God said about Moses and how God dealt with Aaron & Miriam.

> Numbers 12
> 4 Suddenly the LORD said to Moses and Aaron and to Miriam, "You three come out to the tent of meeting." So the three of them came out.
> 5 Then the LORD came down in a pillar of cloud and stood at the doorway of the tent, and He called Aaron and Miriam. When they had both come forward,
> 6 He said, "Hear now My words: If there is a prophet among you, I, the LORD, shall make Myself known to him in a vision. I shall speak with him in a dream.

7 "Not so, with My servant Moses, He is faithful in all My household;
8 With him I speak mouth to mouth, Even openly, and not in dark sayings, And he beholds the form of the LORD. Why then were you not afraid To speak against My servant, against Moses?"
9 So the anger of the LORD burned against them and He departed.

God handled the issue by calling a meeting of the three individuals concerned in the situation. Nobody spoke but God, who spoke directly to the ones involved reminding them of His choice of Moses:

About Moses – Prophet among them
　　　　　　-I shall make myself known to him
　　　　　　-He is faithful in all God's household
　　　　　　-We speak mouth to mouth – openly,
　　　　　　 not in dark sayings

God challenges them as to why they would speak against Moses. There is no response from anyone. God is angry and He leaves. They are not left to wonder what God is going to do next. Read on marking what happened to Miriam, how Aaron responds and what Moses does.

Numbers 12
10 But when the cloud had withdrawn from over the tent, behold, Miriam was leprous, as white as snow. As Aaron turned toward Miriam, behold, she was leprous.
11 Then Aaron said to Moses, "Oh, my lord, I beg you, do not account this sin to us, in which we have acted foolishly and in which we have sinned.
12 "Oh, do not let her be like one dead, whose flesh is half eaten away when he comes from his mother's womb!"
13 Moses cried out to the LORD, saying, "O God, heal her, I pray!"

God departed. Miriam is leprous. Aaron begs! They knew the commands 'listen and obey and I will put none of these diseases on you'. God put the disease on Miriam and Aaron must now acknowledge the same authority he questioned moments earlier. He does not hesitate to admit their sin and ask for help. When you know the verses and are still disobedient, acknowledge the sin, repent and do what you know to do, be obedient to God. Moses, who has not spoken during the entire situation, speaks, not to Aaron or Miriam, but he spoke to God on behalf of his sister. He does not plead his own case, he does not defend her, he simply asks God to heal her. God will heal her, but not until she bears her shame. Read on underlining how she bore the shame and whom it affected.

> Numbers 12
> 14 But the LORD said to Moses, "If her father had but spit in her face, would she not bear her shame for seven days? Let her be shut up for seven days outside the camp, and afterward she may be received again."
> 15 So Miriam was shut up outside the camp for seven days, and the people did not move on until Miriam was received again.
> 16 Afterward, however, the people moved out from Hazeroth and camped in the wilderness of Paran.

Miriam was shut up for seven days outside the camp. All of the people of Israel were at a standstill because of the disobedience of Miriam and Aaron that led to the disease of leprosy, jeopardizing the health of an entire nation. So you can eat all the lettuce and broccoli on this earth, but if you do not handle spiritual issues and walk in obedience to God there could very well be a physical manifestation of your spiritual problem. You may fast and pray and ask for healing but there will not be a speedy recovery until the sin is acknowledged before God. Read the simple prayer of the Psalmist, marking his confession and his request.

Psalm 41
4 As for me, I said, "O LORD, be gracious to me;
Heal my soul, for I have sinned against You."

The Case Against Ignorance

The Bible clearly tells us that we are destroyed for lack of knowledge and God has a case against the people of the land for it. Read the passage below looking for the basis of God's case against the people. Underline the problem as you read.

Hosea 4
1 Listen to the word of the LORD, O sons of Israel, For the LORD has a case against the inhabitants of the land, Because there is no faithfulness or kindness Or knowledge of God in the land.
2 There is swearing, deception, murder, stealing and adultery. They employ violence, so that bloodshed follows bloodshed.
3 Therefore the land mourns, And everyone who lives in it languishes Along with the beasts of the field and the birds of the sky, And also the fish of the sea disappear.

God's case against the inhabitants of the land:

- No faithfulness or kindness
- No knowledge of God in the land
- Swearing, deception, murder, stealing & adultery
- Violence & bloodshed

Result:
(1) The land mourns-everyone languishes including animals and fish
(2) The people are stumbling and so were the prophet and priest. Read verse 6 and underline exactly why the people are being destroyed.

51

Hosea 4

4 Yet let no one find fault, and let none offer reproof; For your people are like those who contend with the priest.

5 So you will stumble by day, And the prophet also will stumble with you by night; And I will destroy your mother.

6 My people are destroyed for lack of knowledge. Because you have rejected knowledge, I also will reject you from being My priest. Since you have forgotten the law of your God, I also will forget your children.

Word Study

<u>Destroy</u> in Hebrew is *damah,* meaning "to be dumb or silent; hence, to fail or perish; to destroy, cease, be cut down (off), destroy, be brought to silence, be undone. This verb depicts a violent end (Is. 15:1; Jer. 47:5; Hos. 4:5, 6; 10:15)".

It was not that the people did not know the truth. They rejected (to cast off, to refuse) what they knew. So someone who does not know the Word of God, out of ignorance or disobedience will be destroyed or cut off violently. As we read on, look at what they feed on. Be sure to mark what will happen when they eat, and why it happens.

Hosea 4

7 The more they multiplied, the more they sinned against Me; I will change their glory into shame.

8 They feed on the sin of My people And direct their desire toward their iniquity.

9 And it will be, like people, like priest; So I will punish them for their ways And repay them for their deeds.

10 They will eat, but not have enough; They will play the harlot, but not increase, Because they have stopped giving heed to the LORD.

Although they eat they will not be nourished and not satisfied, they will be barren because they do not heed the Lord. What is the point? Ignorance (Lack of knowledge) or disobedience will kill you and nothing will satisfy you.

Read the following passage and underline the difference between those who obey and those who do not.

> Isaiah 1
> 19 "If you consent and obey, You will eat the best of the land;
> 20 "But if you refuse and rebel, You will be devoured by the sword." Truly, the mouth of the LORD has spoken.

Word Study

Devoured in Hebrew is *akal*, meaning "to eat (literally or figuratively) burn up, consume, devour, dine, eat, feed (with), food."

Sword in Hebrew is *chereb* meaning, "drought; also a cutting instrument (from its destructive effect), as a knife, sword, or other sharp implement: axe, dagger, knife, mattock, sword, tool."

Those who obey will always be fed and nourished. Those who rebel will be devoured (consumed or eaten) with a cutting instrument, meaning to cut off or amputate. Can you see that the person who is disobedient will experience amputation by their own hand and mouth disease? To be cut off or amputated could apply to a lot of areas, but since the context deals with eating the best of the land I am reminded of those who are diabetic, who will not eat properly as the doctor prescribes and eventually must have limbs amputate. So, what do you think?

When you know the Word and spend time in prayer you can handle the issues effectively. The following passage shows how an issue is dealt with before it gets out of hand, causing additional harm to other people. Read and underline the compliant. Circle *food*.

> Acts 6
> 1 Now at this time while the disciples were increasing in number, a complaint arose on the part of the Hellenistic Jews against the native Hebrews, because their widows were being overlooked in the daily serving of food.

Many people had been added to the early church locally and from all around the country as well. There were no needy people among them and no governmental welfare system. People who owned property, land and homes would sell their goods and bring the proceeds to the apostles who would make distribution as the needs arose. The Hellenistic Jews were of foreign birth and Greek education whereas the Hebrews were native to the area and actually spoke the Hebrew language. The widows of the Hellenistic Jews were for whatever reason being overlooked in the daily distribution. It appears that someone other than the widows brought the complaint. It is interesting to note that the complaint is about food. As you read, underline the decision of the disciples.

> Acts 6
> 2 So the twelve summoned the congregation of the disciples and said, "It is not desirable for us to neglect the word of God in order to serve tables.

The disciples know the issue has to be handled, but they are fully aware that they cannot handle it to the neglect of the word. Read on and mark how the problem is solved. Underline the criteria for those selected to serve tables.

Acts 6

3 "Therefore, brethren, select from among you seven men of good reputation, full of the Spirit and of wisdom, whom we may put in charge of this task.

4 "But we will devote ourselves to prayer and to the ministry of the word."

5 The statement found approval with the whole congregation; and they chose Stephen, a man full of faith and of the Holy Spirit, and Philip, Prochorus, Nicanor, Timon, Parmenas and Nicolas, a proselyte from Antioch.

6 And these they brought before the apostles; and after praying, they laid their hands on them.

The men selected had the following attributes.

Good reputation
Full of the Spirit
Full of wisdom
Full of faith and the Holy Spirit

The men were not chosen because they knew how to serve tables or how to handle people. They did not submit resumes and there is no record that they had previous work experience at the local restaurant. They were chosen because of their relationship with God. Their only assignment at this point is to serve tables. It seems that with all we have studied regarding food and how people respond when there is a lack of food, it is absolutely necessary to have someone that is full of faith, wisdom and the Spirit when dealing with folks and food!

A great deal of emphasis is placed on the apostles not neglecting their time to study the word and to spend time with God in prayer. YES! Handle the issues, but do not neglect prayer and the study of the Word. The apostles in full agreement with those selected, laid hands on them and set them apart for this service. The Word is studied, the prayers prayed, and the problems are aborted because the issues are handled. Read the last two verses and notice what happened as a result.

> Acts 6
> 7 The word of God kept on spreading; and the number of the disciples continued to increase greatly in Jerusalem, and a great many of the priests were becoming obedient to the faith.
> 8 And Stephen, full of grace and power, was performing great wonders and signs among the people.

Results:
The Word and prayer were not neglected
The Word spreads
The disciples increased
Priests became obedient to the faith
Stephen used the table serving experience to expand in other areas.

Don't hinder your growth! It is when we obey God and handle the issues that we can move on to doing great things for God.

The following passage describes a very sick king and how he responded to illness. As you study look closely for what and how the king prays when he finds out about his sickness. Underline what the Lord's message is to Hezekiah and double underline the king's response.

> 2 Kings 20
> 1 In those days Hezekiah became mortally ill. And Isaiah the prophet the son of Amoz came to him and said to him, "Thus says the LORD, 'Set your house in order, for you shall die and not live.'"

2 Then he turned his face to the wall and prayed to
the LORD, saying,

Look at the sovereignty of God as He gives the word that
the king is about to die. Hezekiah is given time to get
things in order, write the will, disperse his property, close
out any open issues, whatever. God gives him that time.
The first thing he seems to set in order is his relationship
with God. Read on underlining his specific prayer. Also
think about what he does not ask.

2 Kings 20
3 "Remember now, O LORD, I beseech You, how
I have walked before You in truth and with a whole
heart and have done what is good in Your sight."
And Hezekiah wept bitterly.

Hezekiah knew enough about God to know that He hears
and answers prayer. So he uses the power and privilege of
prayer. At this point he does not ask God to heal him nor
to stay the hand of death, but he mentions three things to
God:
1-He had walked before God in truth
2-He had walked with a whole heart
3-He did what was good in God's sight
…and he wept…

Read on underlining how quickly God answers the prayer
and to what extent.

2 Kings 20
4 Before Isaiah had gone out of the middle court,
the word of the LORD came to him, saying,
5 "Return and say to Hezekiah the leader of My
people, 'Thus says the LORD, the God of your
father David, "I have heard your prayer, I have seen
your tears; behold, I will heal you. On the third day
you shall go up to the house of the LORD.

What a God we serve! He answers before Isaiah could get out of the middle court and God instructed him to go back to the king and give him the answer. God identified Hezekiah as the leader of His people, acknowledged that He had heard the prayer, saw the tears and promised to heal the king. The healing of this sickness that was unto death would put the king back on his feet so that on the third day he could take care of the house of the Lord. God's answer also came with added benefits. Underline the benefits and the method of healing.

> 2 Kings 20
> 6 "I will add fifteen years to your life, and I will deliver you and this city from the hand of the king of Assyria; and I will defend this city for My own sake and for My servant David's sake."'"
> 7 Then Isaiah said, "Take a cake of figs." And they took and laid it on the boil, and he recovered.

It is for sure that God answers prayer, that He wounds, He heals and that His people have favor. Hezekiah took advantage of the opportunity and power of prayer to talk to God who is in charge of it all. Although God can heal without surgery, medicine or man, He here chooses to use a natural method and instructs Isaiah to put a poultice of figs on the boil and of course Hezekiah recovers. Not only does God promise to heal, but he also adds 15 years to the king's life. For the second time God mentions His servant David with whom God has a covenant to maintain someone in David's line upon the throne. God honors covenant forever! The third benefit not mentioned in the prayer was that God promised to deliver Hezekiah from the hand of the King of Assyria. Hezekiah prayed--what did he get that he did not ask for?

Healing
A speedy recovery
An additional 15 years added to his life

Victory in an upcoming battle

It is not until we read Isaiah 38 that we get a different view of Hezekiah as he talks to God after his recovery. As you read mark what you see about Hezekiah's relationship to God.

> Isaiah 38:9
> A writing of Hezekiah king of Judah after his illness and recovery:
>
> Isaiah 38:16 "O Lord, by these things men live, And in all these is the life of my spirit; O restore me to health and let me live!
> 17 "Lo, for my own welfare I had great bitterness; It is You who has kept my soul from the pit of nothingness, For You have cast all my sins behind Your back.
> 18 "For Sheol cannot thank You, Death cannot praise You; Those who go down to the pit cannot hope for Your faithfulness.
> 19 "It is the living who give thanks to You, as I do today; A father tells his sons about Your faithfulness.
> 20 "The LORD will surely save me; So we will play my songs on stringed instruments All the days of our life at the house of the LORD."

Hezekiah praises God for life, for restoration of his health and for sins that are cast behind God's back. He acknowledges that Sheol cannot thank God; that Death cannot praise and those in the pit cannot hope in the faithfulness of God, but the living absolutely can thank and praise God. Hezekiah did not have the power to cure his illness nor to extend his own life, but he had the power of prayer on his lips and in his heart. So Hezekiah prayed, God answered and this king did not forget to say 'thank you'. Whether an individual, or an entire group, God hears those who diligently seek Him.

The Israelites were in trouble numerous times. In Psa. 107, the psalmist does a summary of numerous difficulties and dangers and invariably calls the people to praise God for His goodness. There were times they were hungry, thirsty, distressed, miserable, and with fainting souls, but the eyes of the Lord was always upon them. They even rebelled against the words of God, but when they cried out to the Lord in their trouble, He saved them out of their distresses. He sent His Word and healed them. Amazing, just a word, a Word from the Lord sent to heal. Healing for the broken hearted, the abused, the rejected, the wounded, whatever the pain, whatever the situation, God has a healing balm in His Word designed as an antidote for your specific problem. A Word sent to heal the broken hearted and to set the captives free. A balm that is so tremendous that if applied consistently will work as preventive medicine. A word that always protects and provides a means of refuge and shelter even before the trouble starts. A word, when believed, that provides peace in storms and peace in calms non-stop. The healing word, the written word of God! The healing Word, the Son of God! The healing Word, living and active! O' that men would praise the Lord for His goodness and His wonderful works to the children of men! Isn't it good to know that God hears and answers prayers?

Psalm 107
20 He sent His word and healed them, And delivered them from their destructions.

Selah – Think About It

1. How can you pray with confidence?

2. What does God require of His people that would cause Him to hear and heal the land? Are you praying *and* handling the issues?

3. How can a spiritual problem result in a physical problem or sickness?

4. How can lack of knowledge destroy a person?

5. What were the attributes of the men selected to serve tables? In what other areas of ministry could these attributes be used?

6. How does discipline relate to obedience?

7. Are you using the privilege and power of God to plead and cry to God for yourself and others?

8. Death cannot praise God and Sheol cannot thank God, are you among the living who hope in His faithfulness and give Him thanks?

9. Can you see why Christians are as sick as everyone else?

Chapter 6

As A Man Thinketh…

Proverbs 23:7 For as he thinks within himself, so he is. He says to you, "Eat and drink!" But his heart is not with you.

A renewed mind leads to a change in our thinking, which in turn leads to obedience in the lives of believers. If we could change the way we think about food, about what we eat, about the harm we inflict to God's temple and the healing we could instill in ourselves there would be an incredible revival in the health of believers around the world. If we could change the way we think about ourselves and line our thinking up with what God says about us we would be well on our way to healthy thinking, peace, serenity, and well-being consistently in our lives. There is a way to change your thinking and it is your choice to do so!

Any good motivational speaker will tell you that the choices you make will determine how successful you are. They will tell you that you can be assured that you will miss 100% of what you never try, 100% of the shots you never take, and 100% of the goals you never pursue. They will tell you that what you think of yourself is the basis of your attitude and what you think will lead to what you do. They will tell you to talk positive to yourself about yourself. They will tell you to tell yourself that you can, that you are able, that you will do it and then instruct you to go do it. They push self-talk and suggest you talk to yourself in the mirror every morning when you arise and every evening before you go to bed. There is great emphasis on what you let into your mind and what you say to yourself about yourself. It is a great idea but it seems to me that God had the plan before we knew what motivational speakers were.

There are numerous scriptures that will absolutely change the way you think about yourself. The Bible tells us what to think on to have peace, what to do when in trouble, in bondage, in need of protection, in strength and weaknesses, fearful, hungry or full, depressed, stressed or blessed. The Bible says we have the mind of Christ. (See "*My Affirmation*" located in the appendix at the end of this book) In Romans 12:1-2, God tells us we can be transformed by the renewing of our minds. Read the passage and underline the action required.

> Romans 12
> 1 Therefore I urge you, brethren, by the mercies of God, to present your bodies a living and holy sacrifice, acceptable to God, which is your spiritual service of worship.
> 2 And do not be conformed to this world, but be transformed by the renewing of your mind, so that you may prove what the will of God is, that which is good and acceptable and perfect.

Word Study

Transformed in Greek is *metamorphoo*, meaning "to transform (literally or figuratively, metamorphose"): change, transfigure, transform. The word implies a radical change. There must be a *radical, thorough* change on the inside (internally) for there to be an external change in our lives."

Mind in Greek is *nooce* meaning "the intellect, i.e. mind (divine or human; in thought, feeling, or will); by implication, meaning:--mind, understanding."

Verse 1 tells us to present our bodies as a living sacrifice. Without reading the next verse we could be led to think that the change is external only, however as we go on to verse 2, we are told that the mind must also be changed. It is clear how to present our bodies and we are told how to change (renew or restore) the mind and that we are not to conform to the world. The result is that we can prove what the will of God is.

So if the mind is changed the action is going to show up in the lives of bodies that have been presented as living holy sacrifices to God! The renewed mind is prepared to understand the Word of God. The renewed mind is moved to obey the Word of God. The good news is that God has written His laws on the minds of the believers and He has provided a resident teacher for us in the person of the Holy Ghost.

He also tells us to think on the things that are lovely, just and pure and we will have peace (Phil 4:8). We are working on the idea of changing our thinking so that our actions will also change. Underline what we are to think about in verse 8 and the subsequent results in verse 9.

> Phil. 4:8 Finally, brethren, whatsoever things are true, whatsoever things are honorable, whatsoever things are just, whatsoever things are pure, whatsoever things are lovely, whatsoever things are of good report; if there be any virtue, and if there be any praise, think on these things.
> 9 The things you have learned and received and heard and seen in me, practice these things, and the God of peace will be with you.

When our thinking is based on the things of God, and our practice lines up with our thinking, then the peace of God will be with us, no matter what the situation is. There is a connection between a healthy spirit and soul and a healthy body. Read the following scripture underlining the connection.

> 3 John 1:2 Beloved, I pray that in all respects you may prosper and be in good health, just as your soul prospers.

John mentions three areas in this prayer – He prays for:

Prosperity of the body
Health of the body
Prosperity of the soul

John seems to tie prosperity and health of the body to the prosperity of the soul.

Word Study.
<u>Prosperity</u> in Greek *euodoo* meaning "to help on the road, i.e. (passively) succeed in reaching; figuratively, to succeed in business affairs."
<u>Health</u> is *hugiaino,* meaning "to have sound health, i.e. be well (in body); figuratively, to be uncorrupt (true in doctrine):--be in health, (be safe and) sound, (be) whole(-some)"

66

As we increase in our understanding and obedience to the true doctrine of the Word of God our soul prospers likewise we will experience prosperity in our business affairs and healing and health in our bodies. It is clear that in order for the body to prosper and be in good health, the soul must first prosper. As our will and the intellect line up in obedience to the Word of God and we follow through in obedience that is when we see the fullness of health and prosperity in our bodies.

In Proverbs we join Solomon talking to His son. He tells him to listen to the words, not let them depart from his sight, and to keep them in his heart. Read verse 22 and underline how the words are described and their relationship to the body.

> Proverbs 4:22 For they are life to those who find them And health to all their body.

Solomon is not the only one that makes this connection. It is interesting that when the prophet Jeremiah predicted restoration for Israel, He says He will cleanse them from their sin, restore fortunes and bring it to health and healing. It is amazing how we strive for health and healing apart from God and the things of God. Anything we get that is not of God is going to be artificial and will not last. Read Jeremiah 33:6 and underline what else God will do when He heals them.

> Jer. 33:6 'Behold, I will bring to it health and healing, and I will heal them; and I will reveal to them an abundance of peace and truth.

Underline the instructions in the passage below and double underline the result in verse 8.

> Proverbs 3
> 5 Trust in the LORD with all your heart And do not
> lean on your own understanding.
> 6 In all your ways acknowledge Him, And He will
> make your paths straight.
> 7 Do not be wise in your own eyes; Fear the LORD
> and turn away from evil.
> 8 It will be healing to your body And refreshment
> to your bones.

Just as we have seen in every other passage, there is a clear
connection between obedience and healing. As the people
turn away from evil God says it will bring healing to your
body and refreshment to your bones. So the promise is
healing and refreshment when the person obeys God. So
the person controls their own healing in their own bodies
by turning from evil and obeying God.

An Example:

Lets work on a passage of scripture where we see healing
and what a person is thinking and how her thinking leads to
action outside the norm. Read and underline the problem,
how long the problem existed and the current state.

> Mark 5
> 25 A woman who had had a hemorrhage for twelve
> years,
> 26 and had endured much at the hands of many
> physicians, and had spent all that she had and was
> not helped at all, but rather had grown worse—

This woman has a 12-year old issue, has spent all her
money to try to get healed and her condition has grown
worse. In Leviticus 15 we find that this issue, this
hemorrhage has put her in a position where she was
considered unclean, as a result she was not to be in contact
with anyone or anything or that person or thing also
became unclean. The priest was to make atonement on her

behalf before the Lord because of her impure discharge. Those that were considered unclean were to be separated from everyone else so they would not die in their uncleanness by defiling God's tabernacle. It is a very real possibility that she has not really been associated with anyone for twelve years and that she is risking her life by coming in contact with others and obviously exposing everyone to her unclean condition.

After enduring for 12 years, being left financially insecure, physically deteriorating and no chance for recovery, she heard about Jesus. Ready for a change, she pressed through the crowd, through the Levitical rules touching people, not on purpose but just to get to Jesus. Read the following verses and underline why she decided to go to Jesus, what she decided to do and what she was thinking.

> Mark 5
> 27 after hearing about Jesus, she came up in the crowd behind Him and touched His cloak.
> 28 For she thought, "If I just touch His garments, I will get well."

Faith comes by hearing and hearing by the Word of God. What she heard erupted into faith and hope that seemed to give her the ability to press through the crowd. This is a woman who heard the word that Jesus was in town and that He was healing. He had been in town and He had healed a man with a withered hand, cast out demons, and healed so many people that all who had afflictions pressed around Him in order to touch Him. She thought that if she touched the hem of His garment she would be healed. It is interesting to note that she did not plan to touch *Him* but only to touch His garment. Wonder if she thought she would defile Jesus by touching Him personally. Read on to find out what happened and Jesus' response, underlining as you go.

Mark 5

29 Immediately the flow of her blood was dried up; and she felt in her body that she was healed of her affliction.

30 Immediately Jesus, perceiving in Himself that the power proceeding from Him had gone forth, turned around in the crowd and said, "Who touched My garments?"

31 And His disciples said to Him, "You see the crowd pressing in on You, and You say, 'Who touched Me?'"

The crowd following Jesus was huge and the press was tremendous, pushing in on all sides. Most knew about His healing powers and everyone wanted to see the next miracle. It did not take long for the healing virtue to leave Jesus and move to the woman, she was healed immediately. With all the people pushing, pressing and touching, it was the touch of faith that pulled the power for healing. Once again her thinking drove her to this action as she pressed through the crowd and touched the hem of Jesus' garment. Read on to see the end, underlining what happened to the woman and what healed her.

Mark 5

32 And He looked around to see the woman who had done this.

33 But the woman fearing and trembling, aware of what had happened to her, came and fell down before Him and told Him the whole truth.

34 And He said to her, "Daughter, your faith has made you well; go in peace and be healed of your affliction."

Obviously Jesus knew who touched Him, but His question and His gaze drew her to come before Him trembling. Without hesitation, she told the whole truth and the crowd heard about her problem and how she had heard of Jesus. They heard what she thought would happen if she touched

Jesus' garment, how her faith had moved her to her destiny and of course experiencing the miracle of Jesus healing her 12 year old issue. She personally experienced the miracle, but the crowd heard and saw first-hand the miracle of healing.

Then Jesus spoke. No rebuke but a wonderful commendation of her faith, publicly restoring this woman who had suffered so much for so long. O' how He cared for her when others had given up on her. She was healed and made well and Jesus said her faith is what did it. She thought about it, moved on it and in it toward Jesus. Her 'issue' was 12 years old! Is there an issue you need, by faith to move toward Jesus? By the way did you notice that Jesus called her 'daughter'? Healing in her body, peace in her soul.

In Proverbs 21:5 what do the thoughts of the diligent lead to?

Proverbs 21
5 The thoughts of the diligent tend only to plenteousness; but of every one that is hasty only to want. (KJV).

It is amazing how distracting illness can be. A great deal of time and money is spent trying to get healed. Visiting doctors, taking certain medicines, being concerned about the side effects, calling for the elders, standing in prayer lines, receiving visitors, as well as arranging for daily care in private homes or nursing homes takes a lot of time and money. There is big business in health care and associated services, from specialty hospitals to drug stores, health plans, diet plans, equipment, you name it, it is out there. These are major distractions from the main course of the Body of Christ.

71

Yes! We should care for the sick. But if there are illnesses that we get because we are not disciplined or not obedient, could this be a major distraction staged by our enemies, Satan, the world and the flesh? Satan is happy when we are not concentrating on evangelizing the world and developing our growth in Christ. The World is happy when we spend all of our money on food, medicines (drugs) and anything that will increase the health of our economy even though it may be detrimental to yours. The flesh is happy when it has satisfied its appetite for whatever it wants whenever it wants it, especially if it looks good, tastes good, feels good, and smells good. Remember the thief comes to steal, kill and destroy. He is winning when he steals our time, our money, and our health. Look at the following verse underlining what the thief will do and what Jesus promises.

John 10
10 "The thief comes only to steal and kill and destroy; I came that they may have life, and have it abundantly.

Word Study
Steal in Greek is *klepto*, meaning "to filch:--steal; take by stealth."
Kill in Greek word is *thuo*, meaning "(by implication) to sacrifice (properly, by fire, but genitive case); by extension to immolate (slaughter for any purpose):--kill, (do) sacrifice, slay."
Destroy in Greek is *apollumi*, meaning "to destroy fully (reflexively, to perish, or lose), literally or figuratively:--destroy, die, lose, mar, perish. Physical death."

Satan was a murderer and liar from the beginning and his purpose has not changed. He used food to manipulate and deceive Adam and Eve and he is doing the same today. Many are taken very subtly, by stealth as sacrifices, literally murdered, dying very premature deaths and many will follow unless we learn to control our appetites, discipline ourselves and press through the mess.

Word Study
Abundantly in Greek is *perissos*, meaning "beyond; superabundant (in quantity) or superior (in quality); by implication, excessive; preeminence:--exceeding abundantly above, more abundantly, advantage, exceedingly, very highly, beyond measure, more, superfluous."

Jesus promises life and that more abundantly in quantity and in quality. The promise is that our lives would be beyond measure in length and in quality (how we feel). The promise is yours in Jesus! The woman with an issue of blood had a 12-year problem and finally she pressed through the crowd. How long will it be before you press through so that you can obtain all God has for you?

Selah…Think About It!

1. How will renewing your mind change your actions?

2. What will eventually overtake us if we always fill our minds and bodies with tasty, but harmful foods?

3. Spend time today thinking and meditating on things that will develop, renew and restore a healthy mind.

4. What is the connection between a healthy spirit and a healthy body?

5. Can you see why Christians get sick like everyone else?

When we are weak then He is strong
We must now realize
Obedience will be the tool
He'll use to make alive.

Obedience brings healing
In body, soul and mind
The discipline to stay the course
Rare treasures one will find
                              E. Ward

Chapter 7

Get It Under Control!

> But the fruit of the Spirit is... self-control...Now those who belong to Christ Jesus have crucified the flesh with its passions and desires. If we live by the Spirit, let us also walk by the Spirit. (Galatians 5:22-25)

A major problem that many of us experience with our eating habits is self-control. Just as with Adam and Eve who could not control their appetite of the flesh and ate when they were not hungry, eating something that they were forbidden to eat, we are doing the same thing today.

An absolute necessity or main attraction at most social events, in and out of the Christian community is food. This old tradition has been practiced since the beginning of time. There were covenant meals, meals at the Jewish feasts and festivals, meals at holidays, meals at weddings, meals at funerals, meals at picnics, family gatherings, graduations, inaugurations, any and most all celebrations, and of course breakfast, lunch & dinner, with snacks in between. Unfortunately we are not disciplined enough to control our appetites so that we do not overeat or that we eat only what is good for us.

The following scriptures will help us see what the Word of God says about discipline and self-control. As you read, underline who is disciplined and why.

> Jeremiah 35
> 1 The word which came to Jeremiah from the LORD in the days of Jehoiakim the son of Josiah, king of Judah, saying,
> 2 "Go to the house of the Rechabites and speak to them, and bring them into the house of the LORD, into one of the chambers, and give them wine to drink."
> 3 Then I took Jaazaniah the son of Jeremiah, son of Habazziniah, and his brothers and all his sons and the whole house of the Rechabites,
> 4 and I brought them into the house of the LORD, into the chamber of the sons of Hanan the son of Igdaliah, the man of God, which was near the chamber of the officials, which was above the chamber of Maaseiah the son of Shallum, the doorkeeper.
> 5 Then I set before the men of the house of the Rechabites pitchers full of wine and cups; and I said to them, "Drink wine!"
> 6 But they said, "We will not drink wine, for Jonadab the son of Rechab, our father, commanded us, saying, 'You shall not drink wine, you or your sons, forever.

The Rechabites had been taught that they were not to drink, so when the opportunity presented itself for them to drink, they remembered their father's command and chose not to drink. Not only do we see them preserving their bodies in temperance by not drinking the wine and holding on to the ability to exercise sober reason, but we also see an excellent example of obedience to their parents command.

Wise parents would do well to make sure their children have a real handle on both temperance and obedience.

Read the following verse and mark the warning and the encouragement to exercise self-control in what you eat and in who you associate with.

> Psalm 141
> 4 Do not incline my heart to any evil thing, to practice deeds of wickedness With men who do iniquity; And do not let me eat of their delicacies.

Do not let the prosperity of the wicked, their fancy foods or anything else lead you to wickedness.

Instructions had been given to Israel about their obedience. They are told what to do and why to do it. They are also told what will happen if they refuse to obey. Read the following passage and underline the instructions and the results of obedience and the results of disobedience.

> Deuteronomy 11
> 13 "It shall come about, if you listen obediently to my commandments which I am commanding you today, to love the LORD your God and to serve Him with all your heart and all your soul,
> 14 that He will give the rain for your land in its season, the early and late rain, that you may gather in your grain and your new wine and your oil.
> 15 "He will give grass in your fields for your cattle, and you will eat and be satisfied.

God tied their obedience to the rain on the land, the fruit of the land, and to the food they were to eat. Read verses 16 and 17 underlining the warnings for disobedience.

Deuteronomy 11

16 "Beware that your hearts are not deceived, and that you do not turn away and serve other gods and worship them.

17 "Or the anger of the LORD will be kindled against you, and He will shut up the heavens so that there will be no rain and the ground will not yield its fruit; and you will perish quickly from the good land which the LORD is giving you.

No obedience = no rain = no food = death! Read the following passage and mark who the King of Israel is at this time, his relationship to God, what he has done.

1 Kings 16

29 Now Ahab the son of Omri became king over Israel in the thirty-eighth year of Asa king of Judah, and Ahab the son of Omri reigned over Israel in Samaria twenty-two years.

30 Ahab the son of Omri did evil in the sight of the LORD more than all who were before him.

31 It came about, as though it had been a trivial thing for him to walk in the sins of Jeroboam the son of Nebat, that he married Jezebel the daughter of Ethbaal king of the Sidonians, and went to serve Baal and worshiped him.

32 So he erected an altar for Baal in the house of Baal which he built in Samaria.

33 Ahab also made the Asherah. Thus Ahab did more to provoke the LORD God of Israel than all the kings of Israel who were before him.

Ahab had total disregard for God and His instructions, doing wrong and provoking God more than all the kings of Israel. So God, true to His Word, took action based on His Word. Read 1 Kings 17:1, underlining God's faithful action.

1 Kings 17

1 Now Elijah the Tishbite, who was of the settlers of Gilead, said to Ahab, "As the LORD, the God of

Israel lives, before whom I stand, surely there shall be neither dew nor rain these years, except by my word."

Elijah has the assignment of informing the king of God's message that it was not going to rain for three years and six months (James 5:17). The king and the people had cast God off, turned to other gods, and were totally out of control. King Ahab led the people in this idolatrous action so God took action to discipline His people and bring them in line with His Word.

> 1 Kings 17
> 2 The word of the LORD came to him, saying,
> 3 "Go away from here and turn eastward, and hide yourself by the brook Cherith, which is east of the Jordan.
> 4 "It shall be that you will drink of the brook, and I have commanded the ravens to provide for you there."
> 5 So he went and did according to the word of the LORD, for he went and lived by the brook Cherith, which is east of the Jordan.
> 6 The ravens brought him bread and meat in the morning and bread and meat in the evening, and he would drink from the brook.
> 7 It happened after a while that the brook dried up, because there was no rain in the land.

The king has been given the news that there will be no rain for years and that there will be a famine in the land. Elijah has a dangerous mission assignment, but God sends Elijah to a safe place and promises to provide for him. The prophet received food from a raven, a very unlikely source. The raven, a ravenous unclean bird, who neglected his young, and was timid toward man was commanded by God to give up his prey and provide God's man two meals a day in a famine starved land. Even in an out of control, chaotic situation, God still orchestrates control. God will work in a mighty way in you to do His good pleasure as you lean toward Him in obedience. Elijah's water source dried up and it was time to move on. God will let you know when it is time to move.

> 1 Kings 17
> 8 Then the word of the LORD came to him, saying,
> 9 "Arise, go to Zarephath, which belongs to Sidon, and stay there; behold, I have commanded a widow there to provide for you."
> 10 So he arose and went to Zarephath, and when he came to the gate of the city, behold, a widow was there gathering sticks; and he called to her and said, "Please get me a little water in a jar, that I may drink."
> 11 As she was going to get it, he called to her and said, "Please bring me a piece of bread in your hand."
> 12 But she said, "As the LORD your God lives, I have no bread, only a handful of flour in the bowl and a little oil in the jar; and behold, I am gathering a few sticks that I may go in and prepare for me and my son, that we may eat it and die."

God sent Elijah to another unlikely source, a woman who has no means of provision, very little resources on hand, is desperate and desolate and announces to the prophet her plan to eat her last meal and die. This widow woman who could actually be the one requesting help does not question Elijah about his position but is clearly aware that the LORD is his God. She does not object to his request, does not complain about her situation or of the famine in the land. She seems resigned to the idea that she is going to die, but obviously God has another plan. Read on and underline God's provision for the prophet as well as for the widow and her son.

1 Kings 17

13 Then Elijah said to her, "Do not fear; go, do as you have said, but make me a little bread cake from it first and bring it out to me, and afterward you may make one for yourself and for your son.

14 "For thus says the LORD God of Israel, 'The bowl of flour shall not be exhausted, nor shall the jar of oil be empty, until the day that the LORD sends rain on the face of the earth.'"

What tremendous provisions God made so that for the next three and one half years there would be food in the house for Elijah, the widow and her son. While God sent Elijah as the vessel of correction and discipline for the king and the people of Israel for their disobedience, He at the same time makes provisions for a Gentile woman. It is apparent that He disciplines and corrects Israel by withholding food, but at the same time He disciplines and encourages a Gentile woman by providing food. In the widow's case: Obedience = food (without rain) = life!

1 Kings 17

15 So she went and did according to the word of Elijah, and she and he and her household ate for many days.

16 The bowl of flour was not exhausted nor did the jar of oil become empty, according to the word of the LORD which He spoke through Elijah.

Somehow, perhaps with hope against hope she does exactly what Elijah requests of her. She moves in obedience, her faith working with her works as she completes the task and receives blessings far beyond what she could ask or think. In fact she does not ask and she is not really expecting to do anything but die. Today many have come to expect the blessing before we walk in the faith and obedience that God requires of us. I cannot help but to think of how this woman denied herself to obtain the greater good. Rather than taking the last of the flour and oil for herself, she chose to deny herself so that in the long run she could live.

Rather than eating up everything in sight what would happen if we denied ourselves today so that in the long run we could be amply supplied with an increase in the oil of God and extended healthy life. What a contrast to Israel and King Ahab who are not walking in obedience to this Gentile widow woman who walks in obedience and is totally blessed when her food supply never runs out.

Read the following passages underlining the warnings and anything that could motivate you to discipline your body and exercise self-control in your eating habits and other healthy living habits on a consistent basis.

> Proverbs 23
> 1 When you sit down to dine with a ruler, Consider carefully what is before you,
> 2 And put a knife to your throat If you are a man of great appetite.
> 3 Do not desire his delicacies, For it is deceptive food.

The instructions in the book of Proverbs cover a variety of areas. Solomon is concerned about eating habits and warns about eating just anything. The idea is not to be ruled by the appetite. What looks good, smells good and even tastes good is not always healthy and good for you. There may be pleasure but little or no nutritional benefit. Read on continuing to underline.

> Proverbs 23
> 6 Do not eat the bread of a selfish man, Or desire his delicacies;

7 For as he thinks within himself, so he is. He says to you, "Eat and drink!" But his heart is not with you.
8 You will vomit up the morsel you have eaten, And waste your compliments.

This certainly puts a different light on "as a man thinks within himself, so is he" when we realize the subject is about eating and drinking. Eating the food of the selfish man could lead to a variety of problems since his heart is not with you. It could present an opportunity to be deceived, entrapped and perhaps plundered. To eat the delicacies of a selfish person will make you vomit and waste your compliments because he has the food and can afford the food, but is insincere and does not really want to share with you.

Read and underline the fate of those who eat and drink too much.

Proverbs 23
20 Do not be with heavy drinkers of wine, Or with gluttonous eaters of meat;
21 For the heavy drinker and the glutton will come to poverty, And drowsiness will clothe one with rags.

Who would ever consider that eating too much would affect your social and economical status leading to poverty and rags.

Talk about eating that will have a long-term impact, read the following passage of two brothers, twins born to Jacob and Rebekah, and record their differences. Mark in a significant way what the Lord tells Rebekah about the two boys. Don't miss her prayer for what seems to be a difficult pregnancy.

Genesis 25

21 Isaac prayed to the LORD on behalf of his wife, because she was barren; and the LORD answered him and Rebekah his wife conceived.

22 But the children struggled together within her; and she said, "If it is so, why then am I this way?" So she went to inquire of the LORD.

23 The LORD said to her, "Two nations are in your womb; And two peoples will be separated from your body; And one people shall be stronger than the other; And the older shall serve the younger."

24 When her days to be delivered were fulfilled, behold, there were twins in her womb.

25 Now the first came forth red, all over like a hairy garment; and they named him Esau.

26 Afterward his brother came forth with his hand holding on to Esau's heel, so his name was called Jacob; and Isaac was sixty years old when she gave birth to them.

Differences:

Jacob   Esau

As you continue to read, mark the differences between these twin boys after they have grown up. The struggle in Rebekah's womb and the differences between these two boys, two nations (Israelites and Edomites) has continued throughout the centuries, differences in custom and religions. Also, mark the relationship between the boys and their parents. Consider again what the Lord told Rebekah about the two boys in verse 23.

Genesis 25

27 When the boys grew up, Esau became a skillful hunter, a man of the field, but Jacob was a peaceful man, living in tents.

28 Now Isaac loved Esau, because he had a taste for game, but Rebekah loved Jacob.

There seems to be some favoritism of the parents to the boys as we see that Isaac loved Esau and Rebekah loved Jacob. A problem waiting to happen, a situation that needs to be bought under control. Mark the word 'birthright' and the details of Jacob and Esau's negotiation.

Genesis 25

29 When Jacob had cooked stew, Esau came in from the field and he was famished;

30 and Esau said to Jacob, "Please let me have a swallow of that red stuff there, for I am famished." Therefore his name was called Edom.

31 But Jacob said, "First sell me your birthright."

32 Esau said, "Behold, I am about to die; so of what use then is the birthright to me?"

Esau is so famished and Jacob begins to negotiate for Esau's birthright. The birthright was the esteem position of the firstborn. Jacob was born holding on to Esau's heel, but he was not the firstborn. Esau was so hungry he was willing to sell his birthright for a bowl of lentils. What is the birthright worth, what is its value?

Word Study

Birthright in Hebrew is *bakowrah*, meaning "the firstling of man or beast; abstractly primogeniture:-- birthright, firstborn."

Birthright in Greek is *prototókia*; meaning "The rights of the firstborn, birthright (Heb. 12:16; Sept.: Gen. 25:32-34). Sometimes *prototókeia*. The birthright among the ancient patriarchal Hebrews conferred upon the eldest son the right of religious leadership (acting as the so-called priest of the family) and promised a double portion of the father's estate (Deut. 21:17) which indicated his authority over the his younger siblings. Thus the firstborn was not only a type of Christ as the Firstborn and High Priest of God, but also a type of Christians as the firstborn who are written in heaven and are partakers of the eternal inheritance (cf. Heb. 12:23). Slighting the birthright was both slighting the high honor of officiating in God's name, and despising that eternal inheritance which was typified by the double portion."

Birthright represented several special privileges for the firstborn male including preeminence in the family. Read the following passage, marking what you learn about the 1st born and birthright.

> Genesis 49
> 3 "Reuben, you are my firstborn; My might and the beginning of my strength, Preeminent in dignity and preeminent in power.
> 4 "Uncontrolled as water, you shall not have preeminence, Because you went up to your father's bed; when you defiled it --he went up to my couch.

Birthrights of the firstborn

1. Preeminent in dignity and power

2. Double portion of inheritance Deut 21:17

3. Assigned the duties of the priest of the family before the Levites were taken in place of the firstborn (Num 8:14-18)

Privileges could be lost - (Rueben lost his birthright because he defiled his father's bed). Obviously the birthright was worth more than a fling in bed with someone, and it was worth more than a bowl of lentils, but in this case Jacob insists and persists and Esau does not resist, but gladly takes the food (appetite out of control) despising his birthright.

> Genesis 25
> 31 But Jacob said, "First sell me your birthright."
> 32 Esau said, "Behold, I am about to die; so of what use then is the birthright to me?"
> 33 And Jacob said, "First swear to me"; so he swore to him, and sold his birthright to Jacob.
> 34 Then Jacob gave Esau bread and lentil stew; and he ate and drank, and rose and went on his way. Thus Esau despised his birthright. (NAS95)

Word Study
Despise in Greek is *bazah*, meaning "a primitive root; to disesteem, despise, disdain, contemn, + think to scorn, vile person."

Esau despised his birthright! He said that his birthright would be useless if he was dead. How many things have *you* given up for the pleasure of the moment? Reputation, friends, family, job, money, spiritual blessings, peace of mind, joy in the Lord, how many things for an appetite out of control? There are certainly many ways that our appetites can be out of control. For Rueben it was women, but, for Esau it was food, and it is food for many people.

It is that instant gratification without a thought for future plans or consequences. Just satisfy me today! Food, that basic need for man that has become feed for greed across the nation.

Many Christians have despised and literally given up the right to be well. Exodus 15 where God reveals Himself as Jehovah-Rapha and basically says if you will listen and do what I command you, I will put none of these diseases on you. But we don't listen; we do whatever we choose to do.

We have given up the right to prosper and be in good health as our soul prospers when we spend more time on physical prosperity than we do on our souls. We have given up our right when we live in spiritual poverty and we do not walk in the blessings that God provides. We have given up our right when we do not take care of these bodies, the temple of the Holy Spirit in living morally, eating, sleeping, exercising, being salt and light on this earth, doing all that God requires, glorifying Him in all areas of our lives.

Look at the warning in Hebrews 12 about this same issue.

> Hebrews 12
> 15 See to it that no one comes short of the grace of God; that no root of bitterness springing up causes trouble, and by it many be defiled;
> 16 that there be no immoral or godless person like Esau, who sold his own birthright for a single meal.
> 17 For you know that even afterwards, when he desired to inherit the blessing, he was rejected, for he found no place for repentance, though he sought for it with tears.

Word Study
<u>Bitterness</u> in Greek is *pikria*, meaning "A "root of bitterness" in Heb. 12:15 means a wicked person whose life and behavior is now offensive to God and

obnoxious to men (cf. Deut. 29:17; 32:32; Rev. 8:11)."

The writer of Hebrews calls it coming short of the grace of God and a root of bitterness. He points out that Esau was an immoral and godless person who sold his birthright for a meal. Esau gave up his birthright and did not seem to have a problem with it until it was time to receive the blessing of the birthright, the blessing of his inheritance. When he wanted the blessing, wanted the inheritance, even seeking it with tears, he was rejected. He wanted the blessing even though he had not done what he should have to receive it.

Isn't that the way we are, when we miss the blessing, when we see it going to someone else, when we realize that we could have had more, then we weep and sob for the right we sold, gave away or trampled upon! The good news is that God is so forgiving.

Read the offer He made to Israel, marking what He asked them to do and how they responded.

> Jeremiah 6
> 16 Thus says the LORD, "Stand by the ways and see and ask for the ancient paths, Where the good way is, and walk in it; And you will find rest for your souls. But they said, 'We will not walk in it.'

Can you believe it? They refused God? God is making the same offer to you today it is your choice! Choose you this day whom you will serve and do it. Read the next passage and you may want to memorize it so that you will remember the importance of running to win.

> 1 Corinthians 9
> 24 Do you not know that those who run in a race all run, but only one receives the prize? Run in such a way that you may win.
> 25 And everyone who competes in the games exercises self-control in all things. They then do it

to receive a perishable wreath, but we an imperishable.

26 Therefore I run in such a way, as not without aim; I box in such a way, as not beating the air;

27 but I buffet my body and make it my slave, lest possibly, after I have preached to others, I myself should be disqualified.

If you intend to win the battle of temperance and self-control as it pertains to eating or any other area for that matter, then you must run not just to be running but you must run to win! It is wonderful to know that when we work to win, that action leads to the ability to exercise self-control in all things. So if you are working on self-control in your eating habits and you are making some progress, you will also see discipline working itself out in all other areas of your life. The application of discipline or self-control rolls over into another area simply because exercising the basic principal in one area moves you to apply the same principle in all areas. We are to run in such a way with a goal in mind, not just swinging your arms around, or making plans that you never put into practice.

Make goals that are realistic, attainable and measurable with a specific start date in mind. You actually have to bring your body into subjection. Verse 27 says buff-et your body (buff-et is to beat into subjection, fight, deny the flesh its desires). It does not say buf-fay your body (buf-fay -all you can eat for $4.99). Prove you are who you say you are in Jesus Christ!

One more scripture please! Look for the benefits of returning to the Lord.

Hosea 6
1 "Come, let us return to the LORD. For He has torn us, but He will heal us; He has wounded us, but He will bandage us.

2 "He will revive us after two days; He will raise us up on the third day, That we may live before Him.
3 "So let us know, let us press on to know the LORD. His going forth is as certain as the dawn; And He will come to us like the rain, Like the spring rain watering the earth."

When the people return to the Lord, He will heal. It is one thing to know what God can do. It is another to depend on His mercy and compassion to totally heal and restore to wholeness. Although the wound is severe, there is always the hope of healing, of grace, of God's goodness and mercy as we submit ourselves in obedience to Him. He promises to come like the spring rain watering the earth. He has torn but He will heal, so let us press on to know the Lord!

Psalm 107
20 He sent His word and healed them, And delivered them from their destructions.

Selah – Think About It

1.   As you read the scripture what was the most significant warning for you?

2.   How does overindulgence in eating and drinking affect your daily life.

3.   Which instruction or warning motivated you the most to discipline your body.

4.   What must you do to win the battle of temperance and self-control?

5.   Are you willing to deny yourself today so you can live tomorrow?

6.   Are you walking in the inheritance, in the fullness of the blessings that God has given to every Christian?

7.   Can you see why Christians get just as sick as everyone else?

Lord I am pressing on to know you
Grateful for strength to walk anew
To prosper in your ways O God
To desire only You.

                                        E. Ward

Chapter 8

Eat Good Food!

*Whether, then, you eat or drink or whatever you do,
do all to the glory of God. 1 Corinthians 10: 31*

What's good and what's not? It could be very confusing. For years the big push was on counting calories. Then we were told to forget counting calories, just watch your fat intake until someone realized we needed certain fats. The confusion continued when we were told to eat a high protein low carbohydrate diet to lose weight, nothing to do with health. Unfortunately this diet turned out to be very unhealthy. So exactly what do we eat? There are so many different diets, grapefruit, South beach, Atkins, and hi-protein/low carb diets. Not to mention diet for your blood type, the food-combining diets, raw-food vegan diet, the 'zone' diet, vegetarian, and fruitarian diets. Each have their pros and cons, some more than others. You name it and it's out there, more than you could ask or think. Notwithstanding all the different diets, most people are on the Standard American Diet (SAD). Basically eat whatever you want, whenever you want it, however you want it, and it doesn't matter how much you want. Jumbo, extra-large, buy one get one free, supersize, 'all you can eat' anything goes! This is not the diet that will lead to good health. So what *is* the answer?

We have tried everything else, let's see what the Bible says. If God created man, the earth and everything in it, surely He knows what is best for us. As you read think about whether this criteria for eating makes sense for you today! Read the scriptures, marking what the Bible says about what was and was not given to eat.

> Genesis 1
> 29 Then God said, "Behold, I have given you every plant yielding seed that is on the surface of all the earth, and every tree which has fruit yielding seed; it shall be food for you;

The basic instruction to Adam and Eve was seed bearing fruit and vegetables.

> Genesis 9
> 3 "Every moving thing that is alive shall be food for you; I give all to you, as I gave the green plant.
> 4 "Only you shall not eat flesh with its life, that is, its blood.

After the flood, Noah was given instruction and permission to eat every moving thing. So in addition to seed bearing fruits and vegetables, animals are included. The exception was not to eat the blood because the life was in the blood. Noah separates the clean from the unclean animals in Genesis 7, taking more of the clean than the unclean animals into the ark.

Word Study

Clean in the Hebrew is *tahowr*, meaning "pure (in a physical, chemical, ceremonial or moral sense):- clean, fair, pureness."

In Exodus God revealed Himself as Jehovah-Rapha and promised to put none of the diseases on Israel that He put on the Egyptians as long as they were obedient to His commands. His commands of course included spiritual, ceremonial, moral, social and health requirements.

In Leviticus God has a clear list of the clean and unclean animals and those He instructed Israel to eat and those they were not to eat. Read Leviticus 11 in your Bible, mark and make a list of the clean and unclean meats. As you are reading and marking, the question is does it make sense for us to follow this instruction today? Record your list in the space below:

Clean	Unclean

Word Study

<u>Unclean</u> in the Hebrew is *tame, (taw-may)*, meaning "foul in a religious sense:–defiled, infamous, polluted, unclean."

Surprising that the simple meaning is polluted and foul. God's distinction between the unclean and clean was that

95

the clean was edible and the unclean inedible (Lev 11:47). It is interesting that research shows that the animals that were called 'unclean' in the Old Testament have been found to be detrimental to our health today.

There are many items on the unclean list but lets look at a couple of examples. Seafood that had fins and scales were ok to eat. Everything else was abhorrent or detestable and not to be eaten. That means shellfish i.e., shrimp, crabs, lobster, oysters, clams, scallops, and mussels. I heard one health enthusiast call the lobster the 'cockroach' of the sea. YUCK! UGH! These scavengers were made to purify the waters by filtering volumes of water removing chemicals, toxins and parasites. As a result the flesh of shellfish is loaded with disease causing organisms making it very dangerous for your health. Catfish perform the same function. I don't think you want to eat what they clean up. When you read Matthew 13:47-48 you have to wonder what the difference is between the good and the bad fish.

> Matthew 13
> 47 "Again, the kingdom of heaven is like a dragnet cast into the sea, and gathering fish of every kind;
> 48 and when it was filled, they drew it up on the beach; and they sat down and gathered the good fish into containers, but the bad they threw away.

Isn't it *funny* that each year our findings are getting closer to what God said long ago? No! It's really not funny!

Another example is what we call 'the other white meat'. Pigs carry toxic parasites, harmful bacteria and viruses that can be passed on to humans when eaten. It has been said that pigs have acidic stomachs and never know when to stop eating. Because of the huge amount of food consumed by swine and the scavenger nature of the food, vermin (worms, bugs, lice, insects) pass through the protective intestinal tract into the pig's flesh along with all the toxins and poisons. So when you eat the flesh of swine all the vermin in the pig embeds itself in your muscle and other places of the human body causing a disease called trichinosis. Not only is swine a danger to your health but read the following passage, noting what God says about Israel and their disobedient practices during Isaiah's day.

> Isaiah 65
> 2 "I have spread out My hands all day long to a rebellious people, Who walk in the way which is not good, following their own thoughts,
> 3 A people who continually provoke Me to My face, Offering sacrifices in gardens and burning incense on bricks;
> 4 Who sit among graves and spend the night in secret places; Who eat swine's flesh, And the broth of unclean meat is in their pots.

We can clearly see the patience of God toward Israel for their disobedience. The people were doing whatever they thought. Rebellious, sacrificing to idols, sitting among graves and eating swine, Israel did not try to hide what they were doing. It is a well-known fact that Antiochus Epiphanes compelled the Jews to eat swine's flesh, as full proof of renouncing their religion. They did so, continually provoking God to His face. Yes, swine were made to clean up the earth and they do a fine job. During Jesus' day they became the short-term home of a legion of demons (Mark 5). Based on what you have read, do you really want to consume the earth's garbage delectably prepared as 'the other white meat'?

Avoid unclean meats as described by God. Stay clear of processed and packaged meat (cold cuts, lunch meats, sausages, and hot dogs) from any animal, clean or unclean.

If you are going to eat meat or fish, eat only clean flesh, organic meat, free of chemicals and growth stimulates. The major thrust of the book of Leviticus is holiness and reflects what God expected of those who had been redeemed. I do know the law was given to the Jews as those set apart for God as a way to teach them obedience and to protect them from various problems and diseases. I am well aware that Jesus fulfilled the law, but please remember all things are lawful, but not all things are profitable. Do you think it makes sense to eat according to God's plan?

In Deuteronomy 12:15-25 God expands the instruction and the people were permitted to eat meat but not the blood. It was to be poured out on the ground. The people were not allowed to eat of the tithe of grain, wine, oil, or the firstborn. They were again told not to eat the blood so that it would be well with them. Remember, the life is in the blood and it is the blood that carries nutrients to every part of the body.

Want to know about other foods in scripture? Read the following verses, recording what the Bible says about the food mentioned.

Deuteronomy 32
13 "He made him ride on the high places of the earth, And he ate the produce of the field; And He made him suck honey from the rock, And oil from the flinty rock,
14 Curds of cows, and milk of the flock, With fat of lambs, And rams, the breed of Bashan, and goats, With the finest of the wheat--And of the blood of grapes you drank wine.

List the foods mentioned:

What a list! If you eat meat, make sure the meats are free of chemicals and organically grown and fed. Read Isaiah 7:14-15 below and 7:21-22 in your Bible where we see the promise of the coming Messiah. Look for food substances, listing them below.

> Isaiah 7
> 14 "Therefore the Lord Himself will give you a sign: Behold, a virgin will be with child and bear a son, and she will call His name Immanuel.
> 15 "He will eat curds and honey at the time He knows enough to refuse evil and choose good.

Foods to be eaten:

When David was on the run from Absolom, Barzillai supplied bedding and various types of food "…wheat, barley, flour, parched grain, beans, lentils, parched seeds, honey, curds, sheep, and cheese of the herd, for David and for the people who were with him, to eat; for they said, 'The people are hungry and weary and thirsty in the wilderness.'" (2 Samuel 17:28-29) Did you notice the cheese?

What about fat?

> Leviticus 7
> 23 "Speak to the sons of Israel, saying, 'You shall not eat any fat from an ox, a sheep or a goat.

The fats from these animals are the hardest fats and will be harmful if eaten. If the fats harden at room temperature avoid them for they could lead to heart disease and a variety of cancers. Ox = cow. Many people have learned to trim the fat. Double-good idea since it has been found that various kinds of chemicals, i.e., pesticides, and antibiotics are stored in the fat. That's not the whole story. Read the following passage for a different, non-confusing angle.

> Isaiah 25
> 6 And in this mountain shall the LORD of hosts make unto all people a feast of fat things... (KJV)

On the first reading, there appears to be a conflict until we examine the definition. This is so good!

Word Study

<u>Fat</u> in Hebrew is *shemen (sheh'-men),* meaning "grease, especially liquid (as from the olive, often perfumed); figuratively, richness:--anointing, fat (things), fruitful, oil((-ed)), ointment, olive, + pine."

Isn't that great! God has this tremendous warning against eating the hard fats and we can clearly see the harm to our bodies. Then He tells us to eat the good fats, like olive oil. God's intention is to bless just as He promised. What an awesome God!

> Deuteronomy 7
> 13 "He will love you and bless you and multiply you; He will also bless the fruit of your womb and the fruit of your ground, your grain and your new wine and your oil, the increase of your herd and the young of your flock, in the land which He swore to your forefathers to give you.

I have used a lot of Old Testament passages and you may be wondering why. Read the following passage and mark any reason you may see.

> Romans 15
> 4 For whatever was written in earlier times was written for our instruction, so that through perseverance and the encouragement of the Scriptures we might have hope.
> 5 Now may the God who gives perseverance and encouragement grant you to be of the same mind with one another according to Christ Jesus,

It was written for our instruction so we might have hope. With the perseverance and encouragement of the scriptures we can have the same mind with one another according to Christ Jesus. Look at one more passage and mark any reason you see to study the Old Testament.

> 1 Corinthians 10
> 11 Now these things happened to them as an example, and they were written for our instruction, upon whom the ends of the ages have come.
> 12 Therefore let him who thinks he stands take heed that he does not fall.
> 13 No temptation has overtaken you but such as is common to man; and God is faithful, who will not allow you to be tempted beyond what you are able, but with the temptation will provide the way of escape also, so that you will be able to endure it.

Again they were written for our instruction and we are to take heed. We are encouraged that no temptation is new and God will not allow you to be tempted above that you are able. But will provide a way to escape so we are able to bear it.

Lets look at a passage in the New Testament that talks about eating. Underline *created, God, foods* and *sanctified.*

1 Timothy 4

1 But the Spirit explicitly says that in later times some will fall away from the faith, paying attention to deceitful spirits and doctrines of demons,

2 by means of the hypocrisy of liars seared in their own conscience as with a branding iron,

3 men who forbid marriage and advocate abstaining from foods which God has created to be gratefully shared in by those who believe and know the truth.

4 For everything created by God is good, and nothing is to be rejected if it is received with gratitude;

5 for it is sanctified by means of the word of God and prayer.

This is a passage that many people believe tells us we can eat anything. Be careful and examine what it really says.

Contextually it seems that Paul is trying to warn Timothy that in the latter days the attention will be on deceitful spirits and doctrines of demons. With consciences seared, they will push the idea that abstaining from marriage and avoiding certain foods will move one closer to God. Notice that verse one says that these are people that have turned away from faith and truth to demons. Verse two talks about the hypocrisy of the people pushing the lies. Verse three is great in that it is clear that these hypocritical demon worshippers are trying to convince those who believe and who know the truth that there is a better way to please God than by faith. He pulls it all together in verses four and five by saying that everything that God created is good. Every thing that God made for man's nourishment is good for that purpose and necessary for human life. So ask yourself what did God make good for nourishment and we have to look at Genesis 1:29, Genesis 9:3-4, Leviticus 11, all the passages mentioned in this chapter and any others where God defines what is good. According to verse 4 nothing is to be rejected. Did you notice the criteria?

1. It must be received with gratitude
2. It was to be sanctified by the Word of God
3. It was to be sanctified by prayer

Most people miss #1 and 2 and say that we can eat anything as long as we pray over it. But what does 'sanctified' mean in this passage?

Word Study
Hagiazo is Greek for *sanctify*, meaning "to make holy, i.e. (ceremonially) purify or consecrate; (mentally) to venerate:--hallow, be holy, sanctify, to set apart."

What then does it mean to be sanctified by the Word of God? Could that mean that what God has sanctified (set apart) is sanctified? And whatever God has already called clean in His Word is still clean? Not for our sanctification for we were chosen by the sanctifying work of the Holy Spirit and we have been sanctified through the offering of the body of Christ Jesus once for all. God's people are 'set apart' or sanctified for His use and in this case food has been sanctified for the sanctified. In other words what God called good is still good and we are to receive it with gratitude and prayer. If God has not called it good in His Word we cannot make it good by praying. Notwithstanding all of this if you do eat something that God did not create for food, it will not move you closer or farther away from God spiritually. No, it will not impact you spiritually, but may have some physical impact on your health. So watch yourself!

1 Corinthians 6

12 All things are lawful for me, but not all things are profitable. All things are lawful for me, but I will not be mastered by anything.

13 Food is for the stomach and the stomach is for food, but God will do away with both of them. Yet the body is not for immorality, but for the Lord, and the Lord is for the body.

Selah...Think about it.

1. Why would anyone consider eating according to the outline in Leviticus 11?

2. What foods according to scripture should you avoid just for your protection?

3. What were some of the foods listed that were good?

4. Do you think it makes sense to eat according to God's plan?

5. Does what you eat or not eat impact your spiritual relationship with God?

6. Can you see why Christians get sick like everyone else?

Chapter 9

Lay Aside Every Weight...

> Wherefore seeing we also are compassed about with so great a cloud of witnesses, let us lay aside every weight, and the sin which doth so easily beset us, and let us run with patience the race that is set before us, Heb 12:1 (KJV)

Are you gaining weight in places you have never gained weight in before? Are you having problems getting rid of those excess pounds? Are you experiencing less energy, tight clothing, shortness of breath, and not feeling your best? David in Psalm 32 asks God to show him His ways and teach him to walk in His paths. Don't you think it is time to follow Him to a place of health and wellness?

> Psalms 139
> 14 I will give thanks to You, for I am fearfully and wonderfully made; Wonderful are Your works, And my soul knows it very well.

Obesity is one of the fastest growing epidemics in the United States and is responsible for more than 300,000 deaths per year. According to the Center for Disease Control, two out three American adults (about 65%) are overweight. Many of us are well aware of the health problems associated with being overweight. Those who are overweight are more likely to develop heart disease, high-blood pressure, hypertension, cardiovascular disease, and diabetes. Other areas of health including asthma, sleep apnea and respiratory problems, strokes, gallstones and gallbladder disease, some cancers, menstrual irregularities and even depression are all higher in overweight and obese individuals.

If what you are doing now is putting the weight on and you are struggling to get it off and keep it off, there is help. The way to lose weight, maintain it and be healthy is to make a lifestyle commitment by changing your thinking, your habits, and your behavior.

Striving for the Prize

This is not just about looking good and feeling good. According to 1 Cor 6:19-20 our bodies are the temple of the Holy Spirit. We have been bought with a price and our bodies are not our own. When we look in the mirror and see a temple in ruins because of our neglect, are we really honoring God? Running the Christian race includes being a good steward of all He provides including His temple. Read the following passages marking *run* or *running*.

1 Corinthians 9
24 Do you not know that those who run in a race all run, but only one receives the prize? Run in such a way that you may win.

Galatians 2
2 It was because of a revelation that I went up; and I submitted to them the gospel which I preach among the Gentiles, but I did so in private to those who were of reputation, for fear that I might be running, or had run, in vain.

What did you learn from marking *run* or *running?* Record your answers:

Hindrances to the Runner

Galatians 5
7 You were running well; who hindered you from obeying the truth?

There may be a number of obstacles to keep you from running well in the race for good health, perhaps--lack of discipline, the temptations of fast food places or even mom's kitchen, the busy-ness of our lives or any number of other things. But when you know truth-do it! For God has given you the ability to live and walk in truth.

Read the following passage and mark *Christ, God, run,* and *so that.* Make a list of what you are to do and why.
Philippians 2
14 Do all things without grumbling or disputing;
15 so that you will prove yourselves to be blameless and innocent, children of God above reproach in the midst of a crooked and perverse generation, among whom you appear as lights in the world,

16 holding fast the word of life, so that in the day of Christ I will have reason to glory because I did not run in vain nor toil in vain.

What to do?   Why do it?

Pressing toward the Goal

What is your goal? Is it to lose weight? Or is it to be healthy? Maybe it is both! What and how can you honor God in all of this? Set your goal and strive for the goal letting nothing get in your way. As you read Philippians 3:12-14 mark *Christ Jesus, lay (laid) hold,* and *lies.*

> Philippians 3
> 12 Not that I have already obtained it or have already become perfect, but I press on so that I may lay hold of that for which also I was laid hold of by Christ Jesus.
> 13 Brethren, I do not regard myself as having laid hold of it yet; but one thing I do: forgetting what lies behind and reaching forward to what lies ahead,
> 14 I press on toward the goal for the prize of the upward call of God in Christ Jesus.

- Paul is discussing his relationship with Jesus. What did you learn from marking *lay (laid) hold?*
- What is the goal and what is Paul's plan to reach it?

Can you use these same principles in reaching and maintaining your goal? Is holiness your goal? Whether it is losing weight or being healthy, never forget that your main goal is holiness. You have been set apart for God even in eating and drinking. Whether, then, you eat or drink or whatever you do, do all to the glory of God. (I Cor 10:31)

Write out your goal in the space below. You may have more than one.

Now that you have your goals written. Write out your plan to reach your goals. Make sure your goals are attainable, realistic, and measurable.

Record your plan to reach the goals:

Short term: (Come on-we have to start somewhere)
Daily

Weekly

Monthly

Long term: (If you want long-term results then make long-term plans that evolve into long-term lifestyle changes.)
3 months

6 months

9 months

12 months

Attainable: Be sure your goal is attainable. Do not plan to run in a marathon next week when your current exercise program consists of walking from the living room to the refrigerator. Keep it real! Explain how your goal is attainable.

Realistic: It may have taken you five months or five years to get in the shape you are in. Don't expect to get in good shape in five days. How is your goal realistic?

Measurable: How many times will you exercise per week? Plan your meals in advance and keep a journal on how well you met your goals. Chart your weight! How many hours of sleep are you getting? How much water do you drink per day? Learn to read your body. If you juice fresh fruits and vegetables, how much do you consume? You could even chart your total liquid consumption. Set up ways to measure and evaluate your accomplishments. See example below:

Daily chart:

Weight

Blood pressure

Total fresh juices

Total liquid/day

Exercise

Foods eaten

Massage Therapy

Hours of sleep

Stripping for the Contest

If you really want to drop the weight, you must lay aside, and strip your life of the things that keep the weight on. Now is a good time to think about what you need to get rid of. There are certain foods you need to eliminate from your diet and certain places you will choose not to frequent in this walk for good health? Go back and read chap 8 on 'what to eat'. Read the passage below and mark *lay, run, and eyes.*

> Hebrews 12
> 1 Therefore, since we have so great a cloud of witnesses surrounding us, let us also lay aside every encumbrance and the sin which so easily entangles us, and let us run with endurance the race that is set before us,
> 2 fixing our eyes on Jesus, the author and perfecter of faith, who for the joy set before Him endured the cross, despising the shame, and has sat down at the right hand of the throne of God.

- What happens when you lay aside the weight (or encumbrance)?
- Describe the attitude and the focus of the runner?
- How are you to run and where should your focus be?

Word Study
Weight in Greek is *ogkos, (ong'-kos)*, meaning a mass (as bending or bulging by its load), i.e. burden (hindrance):--weight.

A weight or encumbrance is not only bending or bulging by the load, but it is also a burden on the physical body inside and out (moving slower, breathing, etc). What other burdens are you experiencing with the extra weight whether large or small. Some have more work to do than others, but we all have work to do. A few of the weights you may want to lay aside would be sodas, sugary drinks, high sugar foods, processed foods, artificial sweeteners and foods that include them, high fat products, white flour products and certainly fast foods. Let me give you a little help with a plan.

Make a list of junk food or real food, snacks or others encumbrances that are holding you back. Be honest!

1.

2.

3.

4.

5.

6.

7.

8.

9.

10.

Make a list of places and people that may keep you from running a good race.

1.

2.

3.

4.

5.

In His strength

You may from time to time get weary, weak or discouraged. Pray and learn to say to yourself what God says about you. Spend time in the Word of God, daily renewing your mind. Behavior modification starts with truth and you will be completely successful in His strength when it is understood that the Word is truth! Read the following passages, mark *strengthens, strength, weary, run* and *wait.*

> Philippians 4
> 13 I can do all things through Him who strengthens me.
>
> 2 Corinthians 12
> 10 Therefore I am well content with weaknesses, with insults, with distresses, with persecutions, with difficulties, for Christ's sake; for when I am weak, then I am strong.
>
> Isaiah 40
> 29 He gives strength to the weary, And to him who lacks might He increases power.
> 30 Though youths grow weary and tired, And vigorous young men stumble badly,
> 31 Yet those who wait for the LORD will gain new strength; They will mount up with wings like eagles, They will run and not get tired, They will walk and not become weary.

Word Study
Strength in Greek is *endunamoo, (en-doo-nam-o'-o)*, meaning to empower:--enable, (increase in) strength(-en), be (make) strong. Strength in Hebrew is *kowach {ko'-akh}*; from an unused root meaning to be firm; vigor, force,

fruits, might, power(-ful), strength, substance, wealth.

What happens to those who do get weary and actually wait for the Lord?

How much can we do through Christ?

Based on the definition of strength and what you learned from marking the word *strength,* specifically what will Christ provide?

An inside job

Transformation starts from within. This is an inside out job and God promises victory through our Lord Jesus Christ (1 Cor. 15:57). Read and mark *God, Christ, Spirit* (and applicable pronouns), *work* and *faith.*

> Philippians 2
> 12 So then, my beloved, just as you have always obeyed, not as in my presence only, but now much more in my absence, work out your salvation with fear and trembling;
> 13 for it is God who is at work in you, both to will and to work for His good pleasure.
>
> Ephesians 3
> 16 that He would grant you, according to the riches of His glory, to be strengthened with power through His Spirit in the inner man,

17 so that Christ may dwell in your hearts through faith; and that you, being rooted and grounded in love,

Working out your salvation is how we live by faith, after we are saved, walking in proportion to God's call on our lives to be holy. At the same time what is God working in believers and what is the result?
What did you learn from marking *Christ* and *Spirit*? How is He to dwell in the hearts of the believer and what happens to that person?

Today we have fitness clubs, spas, gymnasiums, home exercise centers, machines, free weights, resistance training, personal trainers, 1001 ways to exercise and we are working harder than ever before to maintain control. A quick overview of the scripture reveals that there was not a lack of physical activity in the days of the Bible.

Moses who climbed mountains even in old age, eyes were not dim and his vigor was not abated (Deut 34:7) and of course he walked from Egypt almost to Canaan.

Jael was strong enough to pull up a tent stake when Sisera wanted to hide out at her home. It was this weapon of choice that won the battle for Israel. (Judges 4-5)

Deborah, doing triple duty as judge, prophetess, and wife, seemed to have enough energy to join in the battle with Barak against the Philistines in Judges 4-5.

Naomi, Ruth and Ophrah walking from Moab to Bethlehem.

From Genesis to Revelation we seeing individuals running; Abraham ran into a herd to get a calf for his guests (Gen

18); Esau ran to meet Jacob (Gen 33); Aaron ran in the midst of the congregation to make atonement for the people (Num 16); David ran to fight Goliath (1 Sam 17); Elijah outran Ahab's chariot (1 Kings 18); Zaccheus ran and climbed a sycamore tree (Lk 19:4); Peter and John running to the tomb (Jn 20:4); Phillip ran and joined the Ethiopian in his chariot (Acts 8); numerous people and crowds ran to Jesus. Jesus climbed mountains, healed the sick, raised the dead, cast out demons, fed thousands of people, admonished the sinners, encouraged His followers and walked throughout the gospels. Believers are a part of this physically fit group. He shed his blood on Calvary so that we would be set free eternally to have abundant life today.

> Jeremiah 12
> 5 "If you have run with footmen and they have tired you out, Then how can you compete with horses? If you fall down in a land of peace, How will you do in the thicket of the Jordan?

If we cannot endure today, how can we even consider that we can deal with issues when they get worse? The provision was made on Calvary, the gift of salvation including abundant life is yours for the asking. Remember it is an inside job.

The Home Stretch--The Award

Read the following passage and mark *fought, fight, finished, faith* and *future*.

> 2 Timothy 4
> 7 I have fought the good fight, I have finished the course, I have kept the faith;
> 8 in the future there is laid up for me the crown of righteousness, which the Lord, the righteous Judge, will award to me on that day; and not only to me, but also to all who have loved His appearing.

As Paul is closing his letter to Timothy, how does he describe his present and his future?

As you run the race for good health, will you continue? How do you plan to finish well?

A fundamental part of weight loss is exercise. Not only will you see present benefits, but also the quality of your life in later years depends on whether or not you exercise today.

Exercise has some weighty benefits:

- Promotes and maintains weight loss. Additionally losing just a few pounds will potentially lower blood pressure and cholesterol.
- Eliminates toxins in several ways:
  - (1) Through perspiration (get rid of your anti-perspiration-we were made to sweat to release the toxins from our systems)
  - (2) By promoting elimination (bowel functions will increase in regularity)
  - (3) Reduces stress and anxiety, which could affect your weight.
- Provides restful sleep
- Helps keep blood sugar, insulin sensitivity and fat metabolism functioning at a healthy level.
- Will stimulate your digestive system and may decrease your appetite.
- Eliminates the extra rolls and flabby skin.

- You will begin to look and feel better about yourself.

Food for thought…

Incorporate good habits in your life, habits that will glorify God. Get rid all the bad or questionable habits that dishonor both God and His temple, your body. Expect a change. You will start seeing your body change when it is used the way God intended. What you can do:

- Believe you can and then 'do it'.
- Your goal is to make a lifestyle change and stick to it. Don't diet.
- Eat healthy food with plenty of fiber
- Eat slowly and chew your food well. Don't overeat.
- Incorporate juicing in your daily routine
- Exercise-commit to some form of activity every day. The key is to burn more than you take in. Consider prayer-walking as a part of your regular routine. Walk and pray for your country, your church, for others, for your family,for any concerns.
- Exercise your mind- read your Bible daily. Read information about health and wellness.
- Detox- cleanse the body of harmful toxins. Give your body a break. There are many ways to detoxify your body, for example:
  - Juice fasting
  - Eliminate junk foods.
  - Exercise enough to sweat
  - Drink extra water
  - Take detox herbs
  - Get a colonic
  - Sit in a hot tub or steam room
  - Get a massage
- Drink plenty of water daily, but not during meals

- Make wise choices! Consider the spiritual implications of your physical choices.

Psalms 119

133 Establish my footsteps in Your word, And do not let any iniquity have dominion over me.

Chapter 10

Restoration Has Finally Come

"For I will restore you to health And I will heal you of your wounds,' declares the LORD..." Jeremiah 30:17

If you are ready to get it together and wondering where to start then this chapter is for you. Or if you want to change and just need help or a push to get you moving and to keep you going then work on the following points. Just maintaining? Keep reading! If you really want to lose weight and keep it off, or if you want to experience dramatic changes in your health, you must practice the following lifestyle changes.

1. Pray For Self-Control To Be Manifested In Your Life.

Prayer is the best-kept secret in the Christian community. God tells us not to worry about anything, but to pray about everything with thanksgiving and He will give us a peace that passes all understanding (Philippians 4:6-7). We are told that we can be confident that God will answer prayers prayed according to His will (James 5:15-16). We are told that we do not know how to pray but that the Holy Spirit will line our prayers up according to the will of God (Romans 8:26-27). We are also told that Jesus will sympathize with our weaknesses and that we can go boldly to the throne of grace and find grace and mercy in time of need. In John 15 we are reminded that if we abide in Him and His words abide in us, we can ask what we will and it will be done unto us. There are numerous scriptures on prayer and if we would simply pray and depend on God as He says, He will do exceedingly abundantly above all we ask or think according to the power that works in us. All this adds up to the fact that if we pray, depending on God, we cannot miss. And we are virtually in a win-win situation. So… Pray…pray…pray!

Scriptures warns us about potential problems with certain foods and the cravings in our bodies. Mark the problems.

> Proverbs 23
> 1 When you sit down to dine with a ruler, Consider carefully what is before you,
> 2 And put a knife to your throat If you are a man of great appetite.
> 3 Do not desire his delicacies, For it is deceptive food.

Be very careful what you eat. Do not overindulge or be persuaded to eat something that is not good for you. What you are eating may not be what you think it is. Some foods obviously have addictive substances in them so you will eat more, buy more, etc. We all know that many foods may provide momentary satisfaction but in the long run cause problems. What happens to the one who overeats, the one who over indulges or as the Bible says, the glutton? Read the following verse and mark what happens.

> Proverbs 23
> 21 For the heavy drinker and the glutton will come to poverty, And drowsiness will clothe one with rags.

The good news is that there is help. If you are willing God offers a tremendous promise and warning.

> Isaiah 1
> 19 If ye be willing and obedient, ye shall eat the good of the land:
> 20 But if ye refuse and rebel, ye shall be devoured with the sword: for the mouth of the LORD hath spoken it. (KJV)

God has given us the ability to control ourselves by the Holy Spirit. Our responsibility is to submit to the Spirit of God and He will cause us to walk in His statutes and commandments. Read the following passage underlining what happens to those who have the fruit of the Spirit, that is, those who belong to Christ.

> Galatians 5
> 22 But the fruit of the Spirit is love, joy, peace, patience, kindness, goodness, faithfulness,
> 23 gentleness, self-control; against such things there is no law.
> 24 Now those who belong to Christ Jesus have crucified the flesh with its passions and desires.
> 25 If we live by the Spirit, let us also walk by the Spirit.

125

Notice (1) who exercises self-control (2) in what areas (3) the result and (4) the responsibility of the person!

> 1 Corinthians 9
> 25 Everyone who competes in the games exercises self-control in all things. They then do it to receive a perishable wreath, but we an imperishable.
> 26 Therefore I run in such a way, as not without aim; I box in such a way, as not beating the air;
> 27 but I discipline my body and make it my slave, so that, after I have preached to others, I myself will not be disqualified.

Verse 25 in the KJV reads a little different. It says everyone who strives for the mastery is temperate in all things. I like the idea of knowing that when I am striving to master one area that I become temperate or self-controlled in all things. So working on self-control in one area will overflow to other areas. That's encouraging!

2. Confess your failure to God when you overindulge

OK, so you blew it and stuffed yourself. Should have stopped at one helping but you didn't. The dessert was irresistible so you had one of each of your favorites, just a little taste of each. Of course you had to take a plate home for later. Next morning feeling sluggish, a little groggy, and slightly puffy, the memory of last night's meal just doesn't seem worth today's agony. Two days later you cannot believe you could not discipline yourself and you are wondering what got into you other than five additional pounds. When you overeat, don't beat yourself up or waste time feeling guilty. Confess, repent and move on. You have a wonderful helper.

> 1 John 2
> 1 My little children, I am writing these things to you so that you may not sin. And if anyone sins, we have an Advocate with the Father, Jesus Christ the righteous;

Word Study

Advocate in Greek is *parakletos*, meaning "an intercessor, consoler:--advocate, comforter."

God in His sovereignty provides help in a supernatural way, but you are responsible to walk in the ability and strength He provides. You are to be good steward of your body, carefully maintaining God's temple. Designed by Creator God, remember you are fearfully and wonderfully made.

3. Study the Word

Line up your habits with the Word of God. The Bible is loaded with information for every area of our lives including what to eat, how to avoid addictions, how to stay healthy and how to live longer. When we understand what the Bible says we will not be confused about what to do about any issue in our lives including health concerns. For example when the world calls for a high-protein, low-carb diet and the Bible clearly includes carbohydrates in our diets, there is no question about what we should eat. Who would know better than the Creator Himself. Read the following scripture underlining what God promises and the result when we pay attention.

> Isaiah 48
> 17 Thus says the LORD, your Redeemer, the Holy One of Israel, "I am the LORD your God, who teaches you to profit, Who leads you in the way you should go.
> 18 "If only you had paid attention to My commandments! Then your well-being would have been like a river, And your righteousness like the waves of the sea.

When Daniel and his friends were in captivity in Babylon they purposed in their hearts that they would not eat of the kings table and defile themselves (Daniel 1:8). It is interesting that Peter encourages believers to arm themselves to live according to the will of God and not to the lusts of the flesh. He is emphatic that it is past time for pursing a course of no restraints, living in lustful indulgences and running with those who do. Read the encouraging words.

> 1 Peter 4
> 1 Therefore, since Christ has suffered in the flesh, arm yourselves also with the same purpose, because

he who has suffered in the flesh has ceased from sin,

2 so as to live the rest of the time in the flesh no longer for the lusts of men, but for the will of God.

3 For the time already past is sufficient for you to have carried out the desire of the Gentiles, having pursued a course of sensuality, lusts, drunkenness, carousing, drinking parties and abominable idolatries.

4 In all this, they are surprised that you do not run with them into the same excesses of dissipation, and they malign you;

It is the Bible that will tell you about the destruction of those whose god is their belly (Philippians 3:19) and encourages you to observe, not forsake and continue in the Word whether you are asleep or awake.

Proverbs 6

20 My son, observe the commandment of your father And do not forsake the teaching of your mother;

21 Bind them continually on your heart; Tie them around your neck.

22 When you walk about, they will guide you; When you sleep, they will watch over you; And when you awake, they will talk to you.

Believe it or not you have an incredible amount of control over your health through the choices you make. Without a doubt you will always make the right choice when you do it according to the Word of God. Without faith it is impossible to please God! (Heb 11:6)

4. Change your thinking

Thoughts, just like words are powerful. As a believer make it a habit to say about yourself what the Bible says about you. Thoughts lead to actions. Thoughts can also increase or decrease stress and can cause the body to be alkaline or acidic. This is important because an acidic body creates an environment for illness and disease. An alkaline PH body on the other hand deflects disease. Thoughts then can cause sickness or thoughts can heal. Some researchers have said that what we say and think can actually change a person's DNA. Solomon provides instruction to His son telling him to listen to the words, not let them depart from his sight, and to keep them in his heart. Read Proverbs 4:22 and underline how the words are described and their relationship to the body.

> Proverbs 4:22 For they are life to those who find them And health to all their body.

Scripture also leaves no doubt about the value of pleasant words to your health.

> Proverbs 16:24 Pleasant words are a honeycomb, Sweet to the soul and healing to the bones.

Have a grateful and thankful attitude no matter what. God daily loads us with benefits (Psalms 68:19) and He has given us the victory in Jesus (1 Corinthians 15:57). When we change the way we think about ourselves and line our thinking up with what God says about us we will be well on our way to good health. As our thinking changes, peace, serenity, and well-being will consistently be in our lives.

> For as he thinks within himself, so he is.
> Proverbs 23:7

5. Eat a balanced diet

In the beginning God created the heavens, the earth and everything in them. Everything God created however was not for food. Most of the items sold in our local grocery stores have been processed and refined so that there is little or no resemblance to the original created form. Preservatives, hydrogenation, irradiation, additives, chemicals, artificial sweeteners, hormones, natural flavors, MSG, and a list of unpronounceable ingredients all promising to enrich our bodies and make strong bones. With all the confusing information what should we eat?

> Genesis 1
> 29 Then God said, "Behold, I have given you every plant yielding seed that is on the surface of all the earth, and every tree which has fruit yielding seed; it shall be food for you;

Based on God's design eat plenty of fruits, vegetables and whole grains. Be careful with carbohydrates. Carbs provide energy and are necessary for digestion, assimilation, and elimination. Studies show that carbs protects the body against the breakdown of essential protein and may prevent ketosis. However avoid refined carbohydrates such as white flour, white rice, and white sugar. God in most of our fruit items has provided natural sugars to satisfy that sweet tooth. If you eat meat be sure it is clean, hormone and pesticide free. A basic and simple rule of thumb-eat your food the way God created it.

> 1Corinthians 10:31
> Whatever you eat or drink or whatever you do, do to the glory of God.

6. Laugh

Can laughter be healing? Can it be good medicine? Research shows that laughter stimulates the entire immune system, elevates depression, alkalizes the body, balances mood swings and is considered to be one of the most beneficial things you can do. Laughter, happiness, and joy are perfect antidotes for stress. Even smiling releases endorphins from the brain making you feel better. Doctors say that endorphins reduce pain and lessen recovery time physically, mentally and emotionally. Laughter causes the adrenal glands to produce cortisol, a natural inflammatory that is wonderful for arthritis among other things. The medical community is certainly moving in the right direction on this one but God said it a long time ago. Look at the following verse.

> Proverbs 17
> 22 A joyful heart is good medicine, But a broken spirit dries up the bones.

An old friend of mine would say, "God bless your bones'. The problem is that many walk around with dried up bones because they find it so difficult to laugh when trouble is coming at them from all sides. God has even provided for that. He assures us that there will not be anything in our lives that we cannot handle (1 Corinthians 10:13) He instructs us to rejoice in the Lord always (Philippians 4:4). In other words God would have us to rejoice in Him and not in the circumstance or whatever may be going on around us. We can rejoice because all things do work together for the good of believers (Romans 8:28) and because God will perfect that which concerns us (Psalm 138). Go ahead – laugh, God will always leads you in triumph in Christ. (2 Corinthians 2:14)

7. Exercise

The Bible is clear that there is great gain and profitability in godliness for the present and future life. But is also clear that there is profit in exercise and discipline for today.

> 1 Timothy 4
> 8 For bodily exercise profits a little, but godliness is profitable for all things, having promise of the life that now is and of that which is to come. (NKJV)

Most experts suggest that we exercise at least 30 minutes – four times a week. Almost everything works! Aerobics, weight-lifting, gardening, walking or running all work if you do it. Swimming, an all time favorite and a great all around exercise is excellent any time of the year. The best easy-to-fit-in exercise, anytime, anyplace, anywhere and very inexpensive is walking. Walk in the morning when the air is fresh, walk at lunchtime instead of having your favorite dessert. Bypass those close parking spots or take the stairs instead of the elevator. Be aware of your surroundings and take advantage of the opportunities to exercise as a regular part of your day. Don't simply change your eating habits and avoid physical exercise you need both. What you put out (i.e., burn calories by exercising must exceed what you put in (i.e, what you eat). Experts say that a regular, systematic exercise program can add five to fifteen years to your life and in turn to your ministry. Don't spend all your time working out and avoid godly exercise, you need both!

> Psalms 86:11 Teach me thy way, O LORD; I will walk in thy truth: unite my heart to fear thy name.

8. Sleep

The Bible is very clear on how much sleep you should get. Too much sleep marks you as a sluggard or just plain lazy. On the other hand we should pull away and rest. Jesus rested and encouraged his disciples to do the same.

> Mark 6
> 31 And He *said to them, "Come away by yourselves to a secluded place and rest a while." (For there were many people coming and going, and they did not even have time to eat.)

Word Study
Rest in Greek is *anapauo* meaning, "to repose, to refresh:--take ease, refresh, (give, take) rest."

Health experts have long known that sleep deprivation is one of the most pervasive health problems in the United States. This problem is responsible for personality disorders, traffic accidents, debilitating fatigue, memory loss, poor physical performance, and illness. As many as 60% of Americans don't get enough sleep. If sleeplessness becomes chronic, you are shortchanging your body and possibly accelerating the aging process. Yet sleep is an absolutely vital component of good health. Adequate sleep actually enhances your health. Regular exercise, not too late at night, helps you to sleep. Eat healthy! A poor diet can interfere with sleep by causing digestive problems. How much should you get? Every person is different but experts still say a good night's sleep (seven to eight hours) is one of the chief health habits of people who stay fit.

> Proverbs 3: 24 When you lie down, you will not be afraid; When you lie down, your sleep will be sweet.

9. Read – be informed

Contrary to popular belief, ignorance is not bliss! What you do not know can hurt you, in fact what you do not know can destroy you. The meaning for the Hebrew word for 'destroy' is to cause, to cut off, to be silent, to perish. Lack of knowledge will keep you unaware of the dangers you may be exposed to, and keep you from knowing what may be good or bad for you. The worse part is that it can lead to destruction and totally destroy you. The same problem occurred in Hosea's day.

> Hosea 4
> 6 My people are destroyed for lack of knowledge. Because you have rejected knowledge, I also will reject you from being My priest. Since you have forgotten the law of your God, I also will forget your children.

When the opportunity is there, not to pursue knowledge is willful ignorance. In the case of Hosea, the priest had the knowledge available to them and rejected it. They should have known. In fact they did know. They knew the law of God and had forgotten it. How tragic to know it and not use it, to have know it and forgotten it. There is so much information available in every type of media you can think of. Many people know the good and bad about health and nutrition, but choose to ignore it. There are actually some that do not know period.

> Isaiah 5
> 13 Therefore My people go into exile for their lack of knowledge; And their honorable men are famished, And their multitude is parched with thirst.

In this case the people did not know and went into captivity for their lack of knowledge. And so it is today. There are people who just do not know and are in total bondage to various foods and other destructive behaviors that can destroy them. Most people know something, but are not interested enough to do a thorough study even though it is their health and their life. What can you do and where is the information available? Health food stores and libraries are good sources for information. Internet services have an incredible amount of information as well. Christian bookstores or your Church's library are other good sources of information. Read the ingredients on the products you purchase. Be aware of the food additives that are harmful to your health. For example there are so many harmful dyes added to our food today, just to make them look pretty, that they have to be numbered. Read the newspapers and articles in some of your favorite magazines. And please, do not believe everything you read, check it out, then check it again. Don't just go with what the crowd says or what the crowd thinks or desires. The majority may rule, but that does not mean they are right. *More than anything read your Bible.* It is the knowledge of the Word of God that will relieve pain, keep you from being cut off from the real truth, release you from fear, heal, comfort, strengthen, and protect you as well as teach you who God is and how to walk in all His ways.

Everything you do and all that you read and plan to do should line up with the Word of God, your life depends on it! Every promise of God is yes and you can depend on that!

2 Corinthians 1
20 For as many as are the promises of God, in Him they are yes; therefore also through Him is our Amen to the glory of God through us.

10. Don't Give Up

Some say it takes thirty days to establish a habit. That may be true but please remember we are working on a lifetime endeavor so plan to go as long as it takes to get and keep your body-God's temple in the best health possible. We have a lot of work to do in the Kingdom. We are a people 'set apart' and that of course includes our health. Just as we are consistent in our spiritual walk, we ought also to be in our physical walk. Will you ever get discouraged? Probably! You may not lose weight as quickly as you would like; you may not eat exactly right at first, but 'don't give up'! The change you are looking for can only come through consistent practice of eating healthy, regular exercise, proper sleep, renewing your mind and walking according to the Word of God! I Samuel 30 has an incredible story of King David who *encouraged himself* when his good friends and close fighting companions wanted to stone him when their enemies attached their city. Friends and family may not agree with you about what you have decided to do with your health. Don't give up! When you cannot find any one to workout with you, or there is no one to share a good healthy meal with you and you are the only one in the crowd trying to get it together, remember you can do it! When everyone is doing the opposite and you begin to think what you are doing is radical, remember you are more than a conqueror. Don't give up! In the story of the woman that had an issue of blood for twelve years, she spent all of her money going from doctor to doctor but she did not get better, and no one could help her, no one. She heard there was a man in town healing the sick. She made her way to the crowd and pushed her way through the press of that crowd. She believed if she touched the hem of Jesus' garment she would be healed. You've got it, she believed it, she pressed, she touched His hem and the healing virtue left Him and healed her. He called her out and she told her entire story in front of the crowd. Do you

137

know what he said? "Daughter, your faith has made you whole" (Mark 5). When you get weary, and you will, don't give up! When you have tried everything you can think of and there is no one to help, remember the woman with a 12-year old issue who pressed through a crowd to get to Jesus because she believed Him! She was restored completely and made whole by the healing transforming power of Jesus Christ. Whatever you need to do to press through, do it, so you can get to Jesus! There is help! Psalm 46 says He is a very present help in trouble. He is a right here, right now God. Don't worry about the obstacles. Believe Him and walk by the faith He has made available to you. You are who God says you are (See "My Affirmation" in the appendix). You can make it. Don't give up!

Psalm 46
1 God is our refuge and strength, A very present help in trouble.
2 Therefore we will not fear, though the earth should change And though the mountains slip into the heart of the sea;
3 Though its waters roar and foam, Though the mountains quake at its swelling pride. Selah.
10 "Cease striving and know that I am God; I will be exalted among the nations, I will be exalted in the earth."
11 The LORD of hosts is with us; The God of Jacob is our stronghold. Selah.

APPENDIX

1. Lies we believe…& Scriptures to help us overcome!

2. My Affirmation

3. To Desire Only You

Lies we believe…& Scriptures to help us overcome!

1. I don't know what to eat. I feel guilty when I eat a snack from time to time. Food can become your god.

A safe rule of thumb is to eat food as close to the way God created it as possible (Gen 1:29). Eat fruits and vegetables, nuts, seeds, grains, etc., making a high percentage of your intake raw. If you go astray, get back on it. Discipline is key! Remember the old adage you eat to live not live to eat. Food is not to be an obsession, so don't let it rule you, you manage it.

> Matthew 6
> 31 "Do not worry then, saying, 'What will we eat?' or 'What will we drink?' or 'What will we wear for clothing?'
> 32 "For the Gentiles eagerly seek all these things; for your heavenly Father knows that you need all these things.
> 33 "But seek first His kingdom and His righteousness, and all these things will be added to you.
> 34 "So do not worry about tomorrow; for tomorrow will care for itself. Each day has enough trouble of its own.

2. It is too expensive

You will pay on one end or the other. Eat unhealthy and you will spend it on Doctors to fix it, drugs to numb it, cosmetics to camouflage it, anointing oil to soak in it and a bed to lie in. Since you have read this book you know what is right.

James 4

17 Therefore, to one who knows the right thing to do and does not do it, to him it is sin.

3. Complaining about the way it looks, smells, and I just don't like it. I don't even want to taste it.

Food can be made to look great and once you began to eat properly you will acquire a taste for the foods that are better for you. Usually when our desire to be well exceeds our desire for a specific taste, we will eat what we should to have a healthy body and mind.

Philippians 2

14 Do all things without grumbling or disputing;

4. I was not raised to eat this way. Culturally I like my food like my mom prepared it. My family will not want to eat like this.

You mind has been renewed. And you are a new creature. The way Mom prepared food may taste great but may not be the best food for you to eat to stay healthy and be an example and a great light for others to see God. A change in your thinking will change your actions.

Romans 12

1 Therefore I urge you, brethren, by the mercies of God, to present your bodies a living and holy sacrifice, acceptable to God, which is your spiritual service of worship.

2 And do not be conformed to this world, but be transformed by the renewing of your mind, so that you may prove what the will of God is, that which is good and acceptable and perfect.

5. I just cannot do it

Yes you can! Believe God and do it!

Philippians 4
13 I can do all things through Him who strengthens
me.

*6. I'm too busy and do not have time to learn how to
prepare the food.*

Take the time now or lose the time later.

Psalms 31
15 My times are in Your hand

1 Corinthians 10
31 Whether, then, you eat or drink or whatever you
do, do all to the glory of God.

7. I don't know where to start, what is best for me.

There are some wonderful Christian resources that you can
find in your library or health food store. A wonderful
resource and point of contact that I have found to be
invaluable is simply ask God to direct your path.

Philippians 4
6 Be anxious for nothing, but in everything by
prayer and supplication with thanksgiving let your
requests be made known to God.
7 And the peace of God, which surpasses all
comprehension, will guard your hearts and your
minds in Christ Jesus.

8. I have tried this and I don't see the difference.
*Besides I'm not fat, I just retain water. My metabolism is
slow and I inherited it from my parents and I really do not
eat that much.*

You may have been trying to eat healthy for a couple of weeks, but since it has taken most of your life to get this way, it will take a while to reverse it. The good news is you can reverse it. Basically what we inherit is eating habits and recipes. So stop blaming Mom and Dad you can control what you eat!

> Joshua 1
> 6 "Be strong and courageous, for you shall give this people possession of the land which I swore to their fathers to give them.
>
> Galatians 5
> 16 But I say, walk by the Spirit, and you will not carry out the desire of the flesh.
>
> Galatians 6
> 9 Let us not lose heart in doing good, for in due time we will reap if we do not grow weary.

9. Sometimes I get stressed or depressed about my finances or my family or circumstances in my life so I run to my favorite comfort food, besides I just like to eat.

There is nothing wrong with eating. God gave us food to enjoy and to sustain us. It is when we eat that which is not meant for our bodies, foods that will harm our bodies or we eat in excess of what our bodies can handle that we run into problems and may end up sick or a long-term disease. You could say this is a physical manifestation of a spiritual problem that we have not handled. Also if there is undue stress or depression, food is not your strong tower. God is!

> Psalms 61
> 3 For You have been a refuge for me, A tower of strength against the enemy.

Psalms 9
10 And those who know Your name will put their trust in You, For You, O LORD, have not forsaken those who seek You.

Proverbs 18
10 The name of the LORD is a strong tower; The righteous runs into it and is safe.

10. I am fine, the Bible says I can eat what ever I desire, pray over it, and I believe God will heal me if I get sick.

True, all things are lawful, you can eat whatever you want, but all things are not expedient and you have a responsibility not to eat things in excess or things that will damage your body – God's temple. If you see Christians who get sick and are dying like everyone else, what makes you think He will heal you when you are not being a good steward of His temple? So Yes, Of course you can eat anything you want and still be a Christian, you will just get to heaven a lot quicker than some of us!

1 Corinthians 6
12 All things are lawful for me, but not all things are profitable. All things are lawful for me, but I will not be mastered by anything.
13 Food is for the stomach and the stomach is for food, but God will do away with both of them. Yet the body is not for immorality, but for the Lord, and the Lord is for the body.
19 Or do you not know that your body is a temple of the Holy Spirit who is in you, whom you have from God, and that you are not your own?
20 For you have been bought with a price: therefore glorify God in your body.

If…you keep doing what you've always done,
You'll keep getting what you've always gotten!
Don't you think it is time for a change?
Selah…think about it

My Affirmation

I Am a Believer!

I am who God says I am 1 Pet 2:9;Eph 1
I can do what God says I can do Phil 4:13
I will be all God designed me to be Gen 3;Rm 8:29-30
I am not down...I am up Eph 2:6
I am not lost...I am saved Lk 19:10
I am not sick...I am healed 1 Pet 2:24
I am not struggling...I am more than a conqueror Rom 8:37
I am not dead...I am alive Rom 6:8,11
I am not in bondage...I am free Rom 6:7; Jn 8:32
I am not under the circumstances...I am an overcomer1 Jn5
I am not defeated...I am victorious 2Cor 2:14
I am not Poor...I am rich Eph 1:3
I am not stressed...I am Blessed Eph 1:3
I am not disappointed...I am anointed & appointed Jn15:16
I am chosen, holy and adopted Eph 1:4-5
I am forgiven, redeemed and sealed Eph 1:7,13
I am filled with the Spirit of God Eph 5:18
I believe all the promises of God 2 Cor 1:20
I can do all things through Christ who strengthens me Phil 4:13
...because I am a Believer in Jesus Christ & His gospel Rm1:16

I Am a Believer!

J. Wilcoxson

To Desire Only You

Why do we seek so many things
Outside your will, Oh Lord
Distracted by delighted eyes
Our flesh it yearns for more.

What is this thing inside of us
That grumbles and complains
We long for foods of Egypt
Though we bear His sovereign name.

When will our aching souls be fed
Our appetites suppressed?
Our flesh caught up in binding waves
Of disobedience.

Let us return unto the Lord
His voice give earnest heed
Keep His statutes and commands
Our bodies He will feed.

When we are weak then He is strong
We must now realize
Obedience will be the tool
He'll use to make alive.
Obedience brings healing
In body, soul and mind

The discipline to stay the course
Rare treasures one will find.

Holy Spirit, Thou take over
Break me from this binding foe
Clean me, build me, make me free
Your healing touch I'll know.

Give me strength to beat my flesh
To look the other way
To deny myself and cling to you
To do exactly what YOU say.

So enlighten me with wisdom
Give me strength to walk anew
To prosper in the ways of God
To desire only You.

Elizabeth Ward

BIBLIOGRAPHY

Strong, James. The Exhaustive Concordance of the Bible*: (electronic ed.) Woodside Bible Fellowship. Ontario 1996.*

Zodiathes, Spiros. The Complete Word Study Old Testament. *Chattanooga, Tennessee: AMG Publishers, 1993.*

Zodiathes, Spiros. The Complete Word Study Dictionary: New Testament.
Chattanooga, Tennessee: AMG Publishers, 1992.

Zodiathes, Spiros. The Complete Word Study New Testament. *Chattanooga, Tennessee. AMG Publishers, 1991.*

Books and Tapes by Jannie M. Wilcoxson:

Books

Let My People Go
Let Not your Heart be Troubled
Looking for Love in the Wrong Place
Thy Word—A Lamp

CDs and Tapes:

- "Nutrition and Health"
- "So You Say You Are in Love"
- "God's Purpose, My Plan"
- "Knowing God"
- "Jude (Studying Inductively)"
- "Hope for the Depressed"
- "Woman, Have You Been with Jesus?"
- "Forgetting, Pressing, Reaching"
- "Living in the Power of His Resurrection"
- "Word Up: The Power of His Name"

For additional information on tapes, CDs, Videos, or Books contact:

SOUND WORDS
P.O. BOX 2105
DAYTON, OH 45401-2105

www.soundwords1.org